Decisions for Living

Strategies for Making Smart Decisions Throughout Life

by

Gopal Dorai, Ph.D.
Emeritus Professor of Economics
William Paterson University of New Jersey

CITI OF
BOOKS

CITIOFBOOKS, INC.
3736 Eubank NE Suite A1
Albuquerque, NM 87111-3579
www.citiofbooks.com
Hotline: 1 (877) 389-2759
Fax: 1 (505) 930-7244

Ordering Information:
Quantity sales. Special discounts are available on quantity purchases by corporations, associations, and others. For details, contact the publisher at the address above.

Printed in the United States of America.

ISBN-13:   Softcover   979-8-90124-418-0
              eBook   979-8-90124-419-7
              Hardback   979-8-90124-420-3

A WELCOME TRIBUTE TO DECISION-MAKING

Many of life's issues are easy and fun to decide,
While others are as hard as they can be.

You might enjoy meeting some of those challenges,
And try to avoid others as long as you can.

You are proud of the many decisions you have made,
Yet would rather not dwell on others that didn't go your way.

Some of those choices turned out the way you wanted,
While others set you back a lot poorer—yet much wiser.

There is no simple way to make hard choices in life,
Except to try, fail, lose, learn, and take your chances.

No matter how difficult the task might appear to be,
One must take risks and play the game until the very end.

Acknowledgments

The germinating idea for this book began several years ago. It has been a slow work in progress with numerous fits and starts. Plenty of real and imaginary obstacles intervened to delay completion of the project.

The broad outlines of the book continued to take shape gradually. Innumerable discussions with family members and friends helped to crystallize several critical ideas. I also benefitted from reading articles appearing periodically in the Wall Street Journal, New York Times and the Washington Post describing how individuals and families made decisions dealing with the various trials and tribulations they faced in life. Some of those stories have served as models for the case studies described in Chapter V. I remain grateful for this important and invisible contribution.

I have benefitted immensely from the help and support received from many individuals. While the book was in the early stages of development, Tara Dorai read the first draft and made numerous suggestions to improve the presentation. K. G. Vaidyanathan typed and retyped several early versions, each time improving what was written earlier. At one crucial point, the entire manuscript somehow disappeared from view and was slowly brought back to life after many hours of herculean effort. The picture on the last page was painstakingly drawn by Vignesh Vaidyanathan.

My lack of familiarity with using Microsoft Word was ably remedied by Niklas Berry. He methodically and patiently put in place the tables and diagrams as they constantly kept shifting from one page to another. The diagrams and illustrations were prepared by Anand Ambrosi. Without his technical expertise and readiness to lend a helping hand, the book could not have seen the light of day.

During the countless times when I needed to make changes to the manuscript, my Project Manager, Juliana Borreggine cheerfully stood by me and patiently took those requests in stride. I wholeheartedly express my sincere appreciation to the staff of Dorrance Publishing who tirelessly worked behind the scenes to make this Book become a reality.

Throughout the many years it took to plan, research and work on this project, our house was cluttered with hundreds of notes, scribblings, newspaper clippings and other writing material spread all over. My wife Kamala has had to put up with and tolerate the resulting mess. Her constant encouragement, many valuable suggestions and unceasing support helped to make this book become a reality instead of a dream.

Ellicott City, MD
September 2024

A Note to My Readers

Those who prefer to have a foretaste of what this book has to offer can test the waters by reading Chapter VII at first. Written in a 'question-answer' format, it covers many of the major ideas discussed in the book.

A leisurely reading of this book should reveal how your own past decision-making experiences compare with similar cases presented here.

It is my fervent hope that readers will be able to put into practice and benefit from using the wealth of ideas contained in these chapters. Depending on your needs and circumstances, you might be able to find plenty of opportunities to apply them in your future decision-making endeavors, as you see fit.

Table of Contents

How This Book Came About

When I first broached the idea of writing a book on decision-making with a scholar acquaintance, he was politely but firmly skeptical of the idea.

"How can you effectively and adequately describe the multiple and complex factors that enter into people's decisions? It is going to be almost impossible to describe them and do justice to the task. There are far too many compulsions, motivations and ideas floating around and working in people's minds, which are responsible for many of their decisions. It is almost inconceivable that you can articulate them and provide useful guidelines."

I pondered this sage counsel for a while. It was discouraging, to say the least. There was earnestness and sincerity in his voice; he did not want me to waste a lot of time and effort in a hopeless enterprise which he thought was going to end up ultimately in disappointment and failure.

Still, the idea kept nagging at me. I was reminded of what my good old friend John Walgreen had once quipped: "Nothing ventured, nothing gained."

I decided to plod ahead, writing copious notes to myself. I thought about the thousands of decisions I had made throughout my life—good, bad, and indifferent. I ruminated on their contexts and possible motivations as much as I could. I tried to recall the successes and failures

1

I had experienced, and how they impacted the quality of my life subsequently. I thought of the many mistakes I had made or those that I managed to avoid. I wondered about the lessons I had learnt from my lifelong experiences/experiments with making all types of decisions.

The more I pondered, the more convinced I became about the desirability of writing a book on this subject. I had a storehouse of ideas which could be used for this project. I knew such a book would be of interest to the general public. I saw and observed how people were going about making their everyday decisions—not always able to explain their clear rationale, and wondering what would happen to them as a result. It was apparent to me that even some of their major, life-changing decisions were not well thought out. A handful of the really important and critical decisions a relative of mine was about to make were haphazardly and hastily chosen. They seemed ill advised and detrimental to her long-term quality of life and wellbeing! Many other people, I observed, were equally clueless and confused. They were unsure of their priorities. Some were unable to resolve long-standing conflicts that were lurking in the background, and still went ahead, making decisions that could later come to haunt them. A few were seeking advice from friends or family members who seemed equally at a loss or unable to offer helpful advice. I became convinced that I could step in and help people like them if I were to put together a guidebook on decision-making (almost like a cookbook) which could be consulted whenever needed. Let me add that when someone sought my advice, I did offer my objective and unbiased opinion on what I thought was the best course of action or solution to a given problem.

To test and put my ideas into practice, I decided to conduct an Adult Education Class on 'Decision-making Techniques.' About twenty students enrolled in the class and they enjoyed and praised the course, reporting that it helped them clarify many thorny issues. Thereafter I conducted a workshop on the subject at NIST, a government agency in Washington, D.C. This was followed by some public lectures and seminars at Howard County Public Library in Ellicott City, MD. I also wrote several blogs about health and wellness as well as on topics related to family financial management.

Encouraged by the success of these endeavors, I decided to continue with my plans for writing this book. I feel that readers will benefit from the wealth of ideas presented here. I have benefitted immensely from reading the vast and rapidly growing literature of books, articles, monographs, and research reports on this vital subject. I am happy to acknowledge my intellectual debt to them for enriching my own knowledge. It is hard to differentiate many of my ideas from theirs; suffice it to say that all of this accumulated knowledge has now become the common heritage of mankind. I offer them to readers with the sincere hope that those struggling with their own personal decision-making problems may find here many useful ideas to help them navigate those murky waters.

Here I am reminded of the saying "Give a hungry man some fish to eat and he will come back for more; instead, teach him how to fish, and he will never go hungry again."

What People Seek through Decision-making

Health, wealth, peace of mind and happiness are some of the most cherished personal goals everyone seeks throughout life. They are often within our grasp, yet quite elusive because achieving them requires constant, unceasing, and determined effort. When we make any decision, we are choosing one course of action over another. The preferred choice is intended to make us better off in some way by solving an existing problem. When you succeed in this mission, there is some improvement in the overall quality of life. However, the decision may also lead to reducing your sense of future wellbeing, either directly or indirectly. Sometimes solving one problem may lead to creating another, making the situation worse off. This happens because we fail to take account of all the possible adverse consequences resulting from the earlier decision.

So, how can we ensure that each decision leads to the intended beneficial result, while avoiding other unwanted side-effects?

Although there is no magic formula to achieve this goal, it is possible to come pretty close to it if we follow certain steps. The aim of this book is to show how this can be done.

Who Is This Book Meant For

People of all ages need to make decisions of one kind or another throughout their lives. These decisions range from the mundane, run-of-the-mill problems of daily living to the more complex questions concerning educational and career choices, lifestyles, family life, personal relationships, financial issues, healthcare and so on. Being able to handle these choices and coming up with the right solutions based on one's philosophy of life is the hallmark of success. Your quality of life is dependent on the cumulative effect of all the decisions you have made in the past. Likewise, your future physical and emotional health, financial wellbeing, standard of living and overall life satisfaction will depend on the choices you make today and the rest of your life. This being so, it is critical to learn how to make decisions that help you to achieve your cherished goals while also trying to avoid ill-conceived choices that end up with negative consequences. While no one deliberately and knowingly goes about making decisions that jeopardize their own future wellbeing, many of us unfortunately fall into this trap all too often. The unwelcome consequences of many such poor decisions are to leave a long trail of suffering, psychic pain, financial losses, ruined relationships, and general dissatisfaction with life. It is possible to minimize such unwanted outcomes by learning how to make and execute decisions that ensure better results. This book offers a dependable roadmap to those who seek guidance on this vital topic. This is an endeavor worth striving for. Readers can benefit from the wisdom distilled here (painstakingly collected from umpteen sources) and learn how to navigate the daunting world of making difficult choices. The book is designed to inform, educate, enlighten, and prepare you for this important task.

When word got around that I was engaged in writing a book on decision-making, it was heartening to hear comments such as:

Librarian: It was a great pleasure attending your seminars on decision-making. There is really an urgent and pressing need to put together your ideas into a book. The sooner you can do this, the better for our patrons. Indeed, a wider audience can greatly benefit from this endeavor.

Neighbor: I hear you are writing a book about decision-making. I really enjoyed reading your other books. When is your new book coming out?

Student: Professor Dorai, many of us who are in the process of applying to colleges find the task daunting. There are scores of decisions to be made. It is all very confusing and time-consuming, to say the least. Is there a simple, straightforward guide on this topic? If not, can you help those of us like me who are seeking guidance on the college selection process?

Home Buyer: My bank is offering me several financing options to buy a house. I heard you are writing a book about various aspects of decision-making. It would be helpful to know how to go about making this all-important financial decision. I can't wait to read your book. Will it have some hints and suggestions on this topic? If not, can you please include it, even though I must make my decision right away?

Colleague: Gopal, when is your decision-making book going to see the light of day? We all need such a guidebook, especially to avoid making bad decisions. The sooner the book is available, the better. It would be timely and most welcome.

I must add that such remarks gave me an additional impetus to write this book. It was reassuring to hear that this effort would indeed be welcomed by the reading public.

I humbly offer this book in the hope that it would serve a useful purpose in helping people to sort out the various aspects of making everyday decisions. My goal is to help enhance the overall quality of life and personal wellbeing of readers by making sound, smart decisions.

What Can You Expect to Learn from This Book?

Most of us have both the freedom and the opportunity to make many choices throughout life. By making appropriate decisions (as one sees fit at any given time), we hope to improve our overall quality of life. The pleasure and payoff that accompany this freedom also entail costs and responsibilities. Being able to make decisions promotes one's self-respect and self-confidence, in addition to the perceived benefits of executing them diligently. We usually decide with the expectation of some future payoff: whether they be financial, professional, emotional, spiritual, etc. Our hope is that the decision will make us better off: otherwise, we would not make that choice.

The various costs of planning needed to make a decision constitute the other side of the equation. One needs to recognize that some of these costs may not always be clearly visible at first. Indeed, they may be lurking in the background, only to be discovered later. When this happens, you tend to exaggerate the benefits and discount the costs at the time of deciding. Those hidden costs may turn out to be large, sometimes stretching far into the future.

Responsible and smart decisions must include a careful evaluation of all potential benefits and costs, regardless of when they occur. Otherwise, it paves the way for eventual disappointment, loss, psychic pain, suffering and regret. This is especially true when you have no one else to blame but yourself for your choices.

Estimating all the benefits and costs of a decision constitute the heart of what is known as "Cost Benefit Analysis." Its purpose is to try to identify and, whenever and wherever possible, quantity them as best as possible. This process can help to determine why you should, or should not, undertake a proposed course of action. It also ensures that the decision is justified only when all its potential benefits are at least equal to, or exceed, the entire spectrum of costs.

While this principle should be self-evident, it is often ignored or brushed aside by some, resulting in unexpected adverse consequences. The problem is that some of the perceived benefits may be illusory and fall short of expectations. Similarly, some hidden costs may drag on for a long time, unobserved or even unobservable. In other words, overestimation of benefits, coupled with underestimation of costs, can present a wholly distorted picture. Likewise, some beneficial decisions may be cast aside (as unworkable) when their perceived costs are(mistakenly) thought to be excessive, relative to their potential benefits. Actions based on such shaky grounds can naturally lead to unnecessary and avoidable regrets.

The question becomes: is it possible to avoid this bias/distortion from happening? If so, how can you be certain that a thorough "Cost-Benefit Analysis" (CBA) can minimize, if not eliminate, this problem?

In your hurry to decide an issue quickly and move on, you may fail to think through all the ramifications of the proposed action. Rather than 'Decide Quickly and Repent Slowly,' one should strive to do the opposite: 'Decide Carefully and Harvest Leisurely.'

Does this scenario seem familiar to you? Have you had situations where your failure to do a meaningful, thorough, diligent cost-benefit analysis resulted in avoidable pain, regret, and losses? Do you wish you had done 'due diligence' before jumping eagerly into that quick decision?

Chapter by chapter, this book addresses all such questions carefully and methodically. Following the ideas and suggestions contained here, you can confidently embark on your lifelong decision-making journey.

It can be a rewarding task—no doubt arduous at first, often somewhat challenging—but eventually becoming routine and habitual! Indeed, the whole process can be enjoyable, instead of being a drag!

Consider this: Thoughts such as 'I hate having to make this decision' can be replaced with 'I feel good; I know that I made the right choice; I am happy and confident with my decision, no matter how it turns out.'

In summary, regardless of whether you are a novice or a seasoned decision-maker, you may discover in this book lots of useful ideas that are informative, educational, and practical. Even some experienced, veteran decision experts may find some valuable tips and insights here, which may enhance their knowledge and expertise. They can judge for themselves whether the book offers anything new or novel that they did not already know! The author hopes that the potential benefits of reading this book far exceed the 'opportunity cost'—by sharpening and improving your ability to make sound, smart decisions.

A Special Word to Novice Decisionmakers

Readers who are habitually hesitant, tentative, or unsure of what to do—waiting and putting off major decisions (educational choices, spouse selection, job offers, relocation/migration, major investments and so on) will find here much valuable guidance, help and support. I know from personal experience, observations and conversations with friends, colleagues, family members, students and even strangers—that many of them eagerly welcomed and sought guidance from me on matters which baffled them. Such occasions made me realize how pleased and grateful they were when even small, marginal improvements in their decision skills did much to enhance their future quality of life.

By this, I mean they derived much greater satisfaction and fewer regrets from resolving the conflicts and issues they were facing.

Finally, those of you who need some 'hand holding' when facing hard choices, or just 'sitting on the fence' wondering what to do, will welcome this book as a Godsend.

In a nutshell, learning to enhance and improve the overall quality of life by making wise, fulfilling choices is everyone's paramount need. If I can even partly succeed in this worthy mission, I would consider my effort a success. I sincerely hope that this will be the case.

Can Decision-making Skills Be Learned and Practiced?

Undoubtedly: Yes.

Some of the decisions you make can either make or break your life. Whenever we make decisions which turn out to be good, we naturally feel happy, satisfied, and fulfilled. Successful decisions in all walks of life—financial, professional, educational, marital, interpersonal, spiritual—can make us feel that we did the right thing at the right time. Conversely, when those decisions don't work out, we are disappointed and feel poorer in diverse ways. You feel emotionally drained. You wonder how and why the decision backfired or tanked. You agonize about why you made a given choice (instead of the alternative available at that time). Was it due to poor judgment, bad luck, or something totally outside your control—an external event? The adverse results come to haunt you, regardless of their real cause. At times, the emotional and psychic costs of 'poor decisions' can be hard to digest; it is fair to say that when a life-changing decision turns out to be disappointing, it can sometimes play havoc with your life.

Therefore, one should ask questions such as:

1. Is it at all possible to make better decisions by learning and adopting new, improved skills?
2. Is there a school or course of study where one can acquire/enhance such skills?
3. How does one go about this task in a methodical fashion?
4. Are there any reliable sources of information on this subject?
5. What exactly is meant by improved 'decision skills'? How can one realistically gain proficiency in this field?
6. Can such learning improve the odds that the decisions I make in the future will leave me more satisfied, fulfilled, and better off? Can I aspire to minimize future disappointments and regrets?

The answer to all such questions is a resounding "Yes." If this were not the case, this book would not have been written nor would you be interested in reading it.

The importance of decision-making skills has long been recognized, appreciated, and taught in many business and management programs in the United States. It is an integral part of many finance/economics courses. Theoretical models of critical decision situations have been the subject of rigorous mathematical and statistical analysis in academic curricula. However, the subject has not received the attention it rightly deserves as part of the basic curriculum in high schools and colleges. This is also true of "Financial Literacy"—a vital skill for managing one's financial life. And yet as the reader can readily appreciate, nothing else is of as much importance to your peace of mind and wellbeing as the ability to make sound decisions throughout life. Perhaps, more to the point, learning how to avoid making 'bad' decisions constitutes the key to long-term mental health. Decision-making is like any other game in which it is possible to enhance and improve one's skills through practice and constant learning. The tools and techniques discussed here should help readers to feel more competent and better prepared to carry out whatever decisions they are called upon to make.

Early Childhood Experiences/Lessons

Most of you probably learnt certain basic decision skills by observing others. From early childhood, our parents teach us about many of life's coping mechanisms. We observe them making choices affecting all aspects of family life. Dinnertime conversations, family discussions, arguments among spouses, siblings, friends, neighbors, teachers and even some occasional strangers provide ample learning opportunities. Watching how individuals and groups in the neighborhood deal with various 'choice situations' provides another useful ground for young adults to learn. Specific instructions to carry out certain tasks assigned by parents or elders also provide many opportunities to learn—maybe you wondered—what could be the rationale for doing 'this' but not 'that' alternative?

Equally important are admonitions and prohibitions not to engage in certain activities, the reasons for which remained mysterious to you. Children are taught to avoid certain situations which might harm their health and personal wellbeing.

Thus, early training in making sound decisions is provided by examples set by others in positions of authority, especially those who are near and dear to us. They serve as role models and provide broad guidelines for exercising 'discriminating judgment,' the essence of making smart choices later in life.

Other Types of Learning Based on Culture & Environment

Most of us initially learn about what works, or doesn't; what is permissible or prohibited, from the environment and culture in which we grow up. Social interaction, religious instruction and cultural norms dictate how one is supposed to act and behave in different social settings.

In addition, the decisions that didn't pan out—one's past mistakes and failures—can teach us a good deal about how one should make better choices in the future. Remember how you fell out of the bike and got badly hurt while trying to avoid hitting someone walking in a narrow alley? Or lost in a debate for lack of relevant information, while your opponents were better informed? Or couldn't sell all the lemonade you had made and expected to sell (for a nice profit) at the summer parade? Such disappointments and frustrations provide fertile ground for learning. Those painful experiences serve a valuable lesson—how to accept defeat gracefully and move on.

Interestingly, the 'School of Hard Knocks' is probably the best, most effective teacher in this arena. Nothing teaches us about making good future decisions as much as the earlier choices we made, which ended in failure. Those adverse results provide the requisite lessons needed to avoid repeating the same mistakes. Of course, this depends on your willingness to learn from those unhappy episodes.

Often people tend to blame others for what went wrong when their decisions do not pan out. You seek comfort by blaming anyone you can think of: God, the Devil, bad weather, ill luck, or the other guy—but not yourself! Unfortunately, this tendency to shift blame is an example of a 'bad' decision. By so doing, you squander away a golden opportunity to learn valuable lessons from your own poor performance. Human nature being what it is, we are prone to attribute our successes and accomplishments to our own superior abilities or good judgment. When things go wrong, however, one is not so ready or willing to accept responsibility (or blame).

What is your own personal experience in this area? Do you indulge in this 'not very helpful' practice—seeking refuge in the 'blame game'? This topic is fully explored in Chapter V.

A 'Sneak Preview' of Good and Bad Decisions

"People tend to attribute good decisions (successes) to their skill and bad ones (failures) to ill-luck or forces outside their control."

Everyone has their own unique way of making decisions. Some don't ordinarily give much thought to the subject while others ruminate a lot before making momentous and far-reaching decisions. The process of decision-making depends on one's personality and attitude. For most people, run-of-the-mill decisions don't need much thought; they follow a set pattern, based mostly on habits and experience. More important decisions are arrived at after careful consideration of their pros and cons.

Perhaps you never gave much thought to this subject. The irony is that though your decisions will impact the quality of your life, people don't always seem to pay enough attention to how they make those decisions. It appears that a great number of people do what they want to do at any given time, without thinking about the future consequences of their actions. This can lead to unnecessary pain, suffering, loss, and disappointment. As a result, a great deal of resources—time, money and psychic energy—are later devoted to undoing what was done earlier. Take, for instance, everyday decisions about health, education, personal relationships, financial issues and planning for the future.

The saying "No one plans to fail, but many of us fail to plan" aptly sums up this unfortunate state of affairs.

Here are some sobering statistics.

Look at the state of America's health statistics. A lion's share of healthcare expenditures in 2020, amounting to almost $700 billion, was devoted to treating diseases brought about by poor (unhealthy) decisions—overeating, smoking, alcohol abuse, inadequate oral hygiene, and sedentary habits—lack of adequate physical activity.

The weight-control industry generates about $147-210 billion in annual revenues. Note that billions of dollars are initially spent on consuming food and drinks that result in unwanted weight gain and billions more are later spent trying to get rid of that excess weight! Does this make any sense?

Consider smoking. A pack-a-day habit costs a smoker an estimated $3,950 per year. For the nation, the annual cost of treating the ill-effects of smoking amounts to $340 billion, including $170 in direct costs and another $165 billion in lost productivity (NIH's National Library of Medicine).

About 6.5% of the estimated 50.5 million high school students (3.3 million) dropped out of high school in 2014. The resulting lost income is estimated to cost $292,000 per person (Graduation Alliance).

Remedial education too tells a dismal story. Millions of college-bound high school graduates are ill prepared to enroll in many basic 101 introductory-level college courses.

They end up taking 'remedial courses,' costing them an estimated $3,000 every year. These students simply failed to learn what they should have learnt in high school, a reflection of poor decision-making in those formative teenage years. All the money, time and energy devoted to this remedial effort speaks to the importance of good decision-making early in life.

The lack of financial literacy and its undesirable impact on people's ability to make sound financial decisions is reflected in statistics on (1) excessive student debt burdens, (2) increasing bankruptcy rates among the general population, (3) inadequate retirement savings, (4) and even the inability to come up with a modest $400 in savings to meet an emergency—as reported by the Federal Reserve in 2022.

Although no one willingly or consciously makes 'bad or poor' decisions, many folks end up doing so for several reasons. Being aware of the pitfalls, traps and missteps which steer you toward making those subpar decisions can certainly help to avoid or at least minimize such unhappy episodes in the future. Most people fail to recognize that some of the decisions they are about to make are poorly thought out and have a low probability of success because they haven't done the necessary homework. When those decisions don't pan out as expected, they are angry, upset, despondent and try to find excuses to shift blame to external factors. Or they belatedly realize that the decision was a 'mistake.' The foregoing discussion naturally leads to the following questions:

What is meant by a 'good' decision? How can one learn to make good or satisfying decisions while avoiding 'bad' ones? How do you learn to recognize the quality of a potential decision before making it?

First, a simple, short answer:

"Good decisions are the result of careful planning and execution; they don't happen by chance."

This valuable lesson was brought home to George, a novice investor, after losing his hard-earned money in a 'get rich quick' investment scheme promoted by a self-serving broker. George had no previous knowledge about investing in the stock market.

After losing a big chunk of his money, George was determined not to repeat this mistake again. He started asking himself the following questions:

1. Why did I make this investment decision? What was I thinking when I took the recommendation of the broker at face value?
2. Did I have adequate, reliable information to make an informed choice?
3. Why didn't I investigate the merits and demerits of this investment carefully?
4. Is it possible that I acted too hastily? Before checking the track record of this broker?
5. Was I too impulsive, irrational, naïve or greedy?
6. Did I use good judgment? Was I swayed by the broker's persuasive 'sales pitch'?
7. Did I consider all other alternative investment choices that were available when this decision was made?
8. Was this decision made in a hurry (without proper reflection) because of a time constraint? I recall the broker saying: "This opportunity will never repeat if you don't grab it now." I was completely swayed by this emotional appeal.
9. I wish I had considered all the potential consequences of my hasty decision instead of just thinking only about the looming prospect of a quick gain. Did I or could I anticipate the potential for losses?

10. What useful lesson can I learn from this unhappy episode? How can I avoid repeating this mistake again?
11. If I knew then what I know now, what would I do?

George's post-mortem soul searching (review) did wonders for him. His losses taught him a valuable lesson. This was the starting point of his learning curve.

The Learning Curve

Academics are fond of describing how we learn—the various types of learning, the sources from which we learn, and the speed with which such learning takes place. This is illustrated in the learning curve, a heuristic device which summarizes our learning experiences over time.

Figure 1

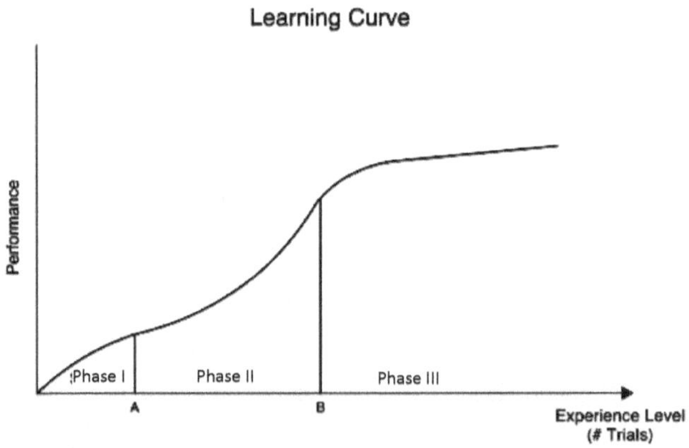

Learning Curve

Phase I: Slow Learning
Phase II: Fast Learning
Phase III: Levelling Off

This curve shows that the pace (speed) of learning is somewhat slow in the beginning (phase I), accelerating rapidly with the amount of time devoted to a certain task and gaining greater experience with it (phase II), and then tapering off gradually (phase III). As is true of most human endeavors, additional units of time spent on a certain activity helps us to gain valuable experiences as well as greater familiarity with it and helps to quicken the rate at which we can perform that task later.

There is no general agreement on the exact shape of the Learning Curve. One may find different shapes as well as interpretations of it. The most useful way to think about it is to look at the many opportunities available for us to learn.

We learn from diverse sources: chief among them being formal schooling, life experiences, observation of others and their actions, as well as from a careful evaluation of the 'mistakes' we may have made in making many previous decisions.

For most people, the first phase of learning is derived from formal schooling as well as from personal exposure to the wide world of different experiences. Thereafter, how much and how fast we learn depends in great part on both the successes and failures resulting from one's previous decisions. Among these, the most rewarding is 'the School of Hard Knocks' or 'mistakes' one has made. There is no greater or more effective method of learning: when things don't work out the way we wanted or expected, we begin to examine what happened and why. When we encounter other people making decisions with which we disagree or hold reservations, we get the opportunity to reflect on their motivations and compulsions. We may be at a loss to understand the rationale for their choices and wonder how we might act when faced with similar circumstances. Likewise, the realization that "if I knew then what I know now"—the benefits of hindsight and broad life experiences—"I would have acted differently" is a common refrain.

Rather than blaming the broker for poor investment performance, George realized that he himself was negligent and should not have jumped on the broker's bandwagon!

In the popular imagination, people interpret 'good decisions' as those which produced favorable results, while 'bad decisions' are those that ended up with negative outcomes.

The 'quality' of a decision should not be judged solely by its results. One must be careful to analyze how the decision was arrived at. There is no guarantee that even a well-thought-out investment decision is going to turn out the way you want. No one should expect successful outcomes always, every time, no matter how much expertise you possess. Even the most experienced, savvy investors know this.

Every decision you make happens in the present, while its consequences—both pleasant and unpleasant—occur in the future. The future is almost always unknowable and uncertain. The probability of making good decisions and avoiding bad ones increases many-fold through a careful, step-by-step systematic review process. Here is a chart illustrating this truism.

Table 1: Types of Decisions (Qualitative Aspects)

EXPECTED OUTCOMES	Good	Bad	Total
Favorable (Success)	60%	10	70
Unfavorable (Failure)	5	25	30
TOTAL	65	35	100%

A 'good decision' is one which is arrived at after careful consideration of all the pros and cons surrounding the given course of action needed to solve a problem. It is based on all pertinent information surrounding the issue.

Notice that when the quality of the decision is initially judged as 'good,' the probability of success is 60%, whereas 'bad' decisions end up with only a 10% success rate. When the quality of the decision is judged as 'good' to begin with, the probability of unfavorable outcomes is low (5%), vis-à-vis a 25% failure rate for decisions termed as 'bad.' (This ratio is 1:5.)

The likelihood of favorable outcomes stemming from so-called 'good decisions' is six times as large as the ones derived from poor decisions. Similarly, but not surprisingly, bad decisions mostly end up with unfavorable outcomes—five times as large as decisions initially termed as 'good.' Of course, even 'bad' decisions can occasionally produce desirable results (10%), just as 'good' decisions can sometimes result in unfavorable outcomes (5%).

To put this in perspective, one should really pay attention to the 'quality' of the underlying decision when judging its results. This is often a 'mixed bag': there can be no guarantee that well-thought-out (good) decisions will always beget desirable outcomes. As Shakespeare wrote: "Virtue is not always rewarded, nor wickedness punished."

This line of thinking naturally leads to the next question: What are the characteristics of good decisions and what practical steps can one take to achieve the expected (desirable) outcomes?

Let me illustrate this with a parable.

Kathy's Marathon Decision

One early September morning, I came across my friend Kathy in our neighborhood park, where she was jogging earnestly. I had not seen Kathy for a long time. I was pleasantly surprised to see her engaged in such serious athletic activity. This intrigued me a great deal. As far as I knew, Kathy was not in the habit of doing any vigorous physical exercise. She abhorred the idea! So, I began by asking her when and why she started her current jogging routine. The ensuing conversation proceeded on the following lines:

Gopal: Hi Kathy, good morning. Fancy running into you like this—a delightful surprise indeed! When did you start this?

Kathy: I recently decided to participate in the 2025 Boston Marathon. I started training for this event about six months ago. To tell you the truth, I got tired of being a 'couch-potato' all these years. I consulted a health pro about how to prepare for the marathon. She advised me to start daily jogging (as a start) for at least one hour every day, gradually increasing the pace slowly and the duration as well—longer by a few minutes. I know I am making steady progress. I can already run a mile in less than fifteen minutes—not bad for someone who never tried this before. I want to build up my stamina and physical endurance for the upcoming marathon. I don't expect to complete the race the first time, but perhaps—next year. I hope to, God willing. I think I can, based on all the effort I am putting into this. I just wanted to challenge myself and see how far I can go. Realistically, even if I cannot do the full distance the first time, I will try again next year. I am determined to complete the race, no matter how long it takes. That is my goal.

Gopal: I am glad to hear that you want to participate in the marathon. How did you arrive at this decision? What inspired you? If I may say so, I did not expect this, and I am truly surprised. Your determination and commitment amaze me.

Kathy: Yes, I understand. I was motivated to try this after watching many runners much older than me. Last year, I noticed that even people with serious handicaps were participating in the marathon, albeit joyfully! Or just for the fun of it, I suppose. They enjoyed the experience and the exhilaration that goes with a great challenge. There was a lady about 75 years old, who relished it. I could not believe my eyes. I thought to myself: If these folks can participate in the race, why can't I? Besides, it should help me to get into better physical and mental shape—I could lose some unneeded pounds, don't you agree? Who knows, perhaps this will even help me to cope much better with my perennial breathing problems. My doctor has been telling me to get some fresh air into my lungs every day, to reduce the severity of the asthma. I may even be able to cut down on my medications and save money in the process. So that is an additional bonus, don't you think?

Gopal: Yes indeed, Kathy. I am impressed by your sound reasoning. You certainly have a strong commitment to this plan. I applaud your decision wholeheartedly. I know that participating in the marathon is really a life-changing experience. But tell me, Kathy, how are you going to manage the expenses associated with this project? I have heard that there are some hefty fees to be paid for admission to the race. In addition, there are also other expenses like travel, lodging and athletic shoes that cost quite a bundle. How are you going to generate the necessary funds? All those items can run into a couple of thousand dollars at a minimum, won't they?

Kathy: Glad that you asked. I did think of that as well. I have asked my mother to help me organize a Halloween bake sale, coming up soon. I hope to raise a few hundred bucks from that. I also plan to start a marathon fund drive. I will solicit help from friends, well-wishers, neighbors, college classmates and colleagues at work—anyone willing to pitch in. I'm even thinking of setting up donation boxes at the local 'Y' and the Senior Athletic Club, where I am a member. Right now, I am in the process of preparing a blog/newsletter, which I will distribute next month among prospective donors. I plan to use my Facebook and Twitter contacts too: I think that would supplement what I can come up with from the other sources.

All in all, I am confident that I will be able to raise a good part of the funds needed. Besides, I plan to look at my current spending habits very carefully. I will cut down my frequent visits to the shopping mall. In addition, I will give up my afternoon Starbucks latte habit. I calculated that this alone will easily free up about $400 by the time the marathon rolls around. Earlier, I had been splurging more than I should have—on things like weekend parties, eating out with friends, and seeing newly released movies. I realize that I must curtail some of these expenses, or even completely give them up. It is all a matter of re-ordering your priorities, I must say. I am determined to be more frugal. I estimate that I will be able to cut my monthly budget to free up about $120 without too much hardship.

Believe me, I don't want to sound like a hermit, but these are the things I must do—no matter how difficult—because the marathon is my highest priority right now. I am eagerly looking forward to it, my friend.

I also have another idea that I will share with you. I plan to increase my contributions to the newly started 'Employee Savings Plan' at the Office. I was putting $50 into that fund every month. I will raise it to $75, starting next month. This savings account is meant for meeting unexpected expenses (some of my friends use it for holiday/vacation spending too). I will build up my kitty for the marathon. So, you see, I have a definite, workable plan, which will see me through.

If you don't mind, may I hope and request that you too will want to pitch in a few bucks for a good cause?

Gopal: Most certainly, Kathy. I am more than happy to do so. I can get some additional financial support for you by asking for donations from my friends and colleagues. I will tell them about your plans—this noble cause. I am confident that they will want to help. We need each other's support, to be sure. I still have another concern about this, though. I hope you won't mind if I ask?

Kathy: What is it, Gopal? Go ahead and ask me. I am eager to get your valuable input and advice. Your opinion means a great deal to me.

Gopal: I know that participating in the marathon is no piece of cake! It requires lots of time to devote to daily practice and sticking to a rigorous running schedule. You are a busy person, with plenty of other social projects going on—volunteering activities, as well as frequent job-related travels. In addition, you have the usual family responsibilities. How will you ever find the time to do all this, plus the strenuous preparation needed for the upcoming marathon?

Kathy: You are indeed very thoughtful, my friend. You are right about those concerns. Thank you for bringing that up. Sure, finding the time needed to devote to the marathon—the daily running regimen—will be tough. I need to selectively cut down on my professional and social obligations. It is not going to be easy, I know. I must make some hard adjustments, some difficult choices, to make this plan work. My family members are supportive, and they will do whatever they can to help with the household chores. Every one of them has promised to help; I consider myself very fortunate in that respect.

So, I think I can handle this problem with a reasonable degree of success. I am going to make a few lifestyle changes right away. I will give it my best shot. With the added encouragement and help of good friends like you, I know I can pull this off. With your kind permission, may I now resume my jogging? I will see you soon.

Gopal: Very well, Kathy. Godspeed to you.

Comments: As the observant reader will notice, Kathy's plan to take part in the marathon demonstrates the essential features of a good, well-thought-out decision. They include:

i) Clarity in formulating the goal.
ii) Adequate planning and preparation.
iii) Finding resources to execute the mission.
iv) Commitment, discipline, and patience.

v) Recognition of potential hurdles—with a workable plan to overcome them.

vi) A time limit to complete the project.

vii) Careful evaluation of all associated costs and benefits

viii) Re-ordering of priorities and willingness to accept the necessary sacrifices—in a realistic manner.

Before concluding this chapter, I would like to dwell on a related topic, which is both interesting and instructive.

"The Inconvenience is Temporary: but the Improvement is Permanent"

The wisdom contained in this phrase is indeed priceless. I noticed the quote on a Billboard while driving along the New York Thruway some time back.

The highway was being repaired and repaved. Severe winter weather and heavy salting to deal with icy road conditions had left the thruway in disrepair. The resulting traffic jams stretched for miles ahead; vehicles were backed up as far as one could see on the horizon! Some motorists were visibly irritated and showing their impatience. Overheated cars and trucks clogged the pavements too. It was a dire situation that had to be endured by everyone on the road.

My friend commented: "No pain; no gain. 'Swallow the bitter medicine, if you want to get better.'"

This remark taught me a great deal about decision-making and left an indelible impression on my mind.

If you want to accomplish something worthwhile, there is a price to be paid; you must decide whether the eventual benefits justify the cost.

Kathy's marathon decision aptly illustrates this point. Her sense of purpose, willingness to accept 'trade-offs,' and put herself through many temporary hardships (while focused on her stated goal) were noteworthy. She knew exactly what she wanted to do, and the steps needed to achieve that mission. Almost nothing was left out of the equation. Careful planning and preparation for the project, step by step, was the hallmark of her vision. She anticipated the many problems, difficulties, and obstacles she would encounter; she was prepared for them and knew how to deal with them. She had a definite, workable strategy to overcome those roadblocks, one by one. She provides us with a concrete, real-life example of what a smart decision would look like.

It is certain that barring unforeseen circumstances, Kathy would be successful in carrying out her decision and reach her cherished goal.

Other factors to consider:
a) **Decisions are influenced by things you cannot control—though they often greatly influence the outcome of your decisions. They are:**
   1. The weather
   2. Political changes
   3. External events
   4. Other people's behavior
   5. Financial market gyrations

b) **Here are things within your control. It is best to concentrate on them to reach your goals.**
   1. Your own behavior
   2. How you choose to react to other's actions or comments
   3. Taking care of your health

4. Be 'proactive' rather than 'reactive' to prevent expensive costs and repairs.
5. Make sensible choices, after careful analysis of issues.
6. Adjust your beliefs so as not to be victimized by 'false' superstitions.
7. Try to get rid of unhelpful habits that could harm you, especially those that prevent you from achieving your goals.
8. Try to take control of tricky situations that happen; use good judgment; don't be alarmed by passing events.
9. Try to balance runaway emotions with a judicious blend of reason. Don't be swayed by others' opinions or actions; trust yourself.
10. Don't emulate celebrities or those in 'authority' blindly.

c) **Gaps in the timeframe of making decisions**

It is often the case that some time will inevitably elapse between the emergence of a 'problem' and the 'reaction time' needed to effectively deal with it. (Look back to your own life for episodes where the length of this gap played a crucial role—for example, a health issue or a financial setback.)

1. Recognition of the problem (after a problem emerges, it takes time to realize exactly what happened and why)
2. Pondering what action is needed and appropriate to deal with it? When is the right time act?
3. Making the decision—Some time will elapse between gathering the needed information and taking appropriate action.
4. Implementing it—overcoming obstacles and doing what is necessary
5. Waiting for results
6. Review and evaluation.

This process is both useful and educative. Looking back on a major decision you made will help to improve your decision-making skills. This provides an opportunity to learn from experience—what you did or didn't do right, how to improve upon that performance in the future. The following questions will help to address this issue.

1. What was the problem you faced? How did it come about? Was it brought about by previous actions you had taken to solve a problem? Or something completely new and unexpected?

2. Did you carefully ponder what to do next? Did you have all the facts and information necessary to make an informed decision?

3. Did you ask for, and receive, any input/advice from others? Or did you feel confident that you could take the necessary remedial action on your own?

4. Did you look at all the available options to address the problem? Did this process involve a great deal of time, money, energy, and skills to collect the requisite data? Did you conduct a careful cost-benefit evaluation of the most desirable option?

5. Were you satisfied that the solution you picked was the best, most appropriate one? Were you reasonably confident that it would work?

6. Did you implement the decision with gusto, and without reservations? Or was it just a temporary stop-gap solution?

7. What happened? Did the decision work out as expected? Did the expected results materialize? Was the problem solved to your satisfaction? If not, why not?

8. Do you need to revisit this problem again? Are you satisfied that the realized results justified the action you took?

9. What can you learn from this experience? How will it contribute to your understanding and expertise in solving similar problems in the future?

10. Do you feel proud and happy that you accomplished what you wanted? Or sad and disappointed that your decision did not work out? If the latter, how would you deal with the problem, if it presented itself again?

This exercise should strengthen your ability to make good decisions and avoid/minimize mistakes/regrets.

The Quest for Accomplishments

Everyone is interested and engaged in a constant quest to improve their quality of life. The question of what constitutes a good quality of life depends on many factors such as age, sex, circumstances, education, personality, values, and aspirations. People generally compare themselves with those they know, such as their classmates, neighbors, colleagues, friends, or extended family members. Regardless of how rich or poor you are, you tend to evaluate and compare your situation with others—this is a game of trying to figure out where you stand in relation to others. Your relative position in the social hierarchy is carefully considered, not in an absolute sense but in relative terms. This is because everyone gets used to their station in life (regardless of how well off you are) knowing that they can work and move toward a more satisfactory position—which is what striving to improve and become better-off implies.

Yet there are certain basic and important constituents that define one's quality of life. These are:

1. Good physical health—the ability to perform all bodily functions satisfactorily.
2. Mental/psychological/emotional health: Freedom from excessive stress, worry, anxiety and tension.
3. A good source of livelihood (steady flow of income) that provides an adequate standard of living.
4. Emotionally satisfying and stable relationships that contribute to feelings of belonging, love, comfort, and personal satisfaction.
5. Feelings of security and confidence.
6. Peace of mind and having a sense of control that you can handle your destiny (within limits).

To secure these, one must be able to make decisions and take actions that promote the quality of life you aspire to. To do so effectively, you must know your strengths and weaknesses.

Anatomy of a Decision: A Parable

Imagine your life in a vast, sprawling multi-storied mansion with many rooms, located on different floors. Some of the rooms are large, while others are small. There are umpteen staircases, nooks and corners, each one different in size, shape and location, spread throughout the mansion. Some of these are easy to locate, while others are hard to find.

You have been assigned the task of painting, repairing, remodeling, furnishing, and decorating the entire mansion. Several rooms have high ceilings and large windows, allowing plenty of sunlight to stream in. Others are narrow and dingy. A few of them allow very little or almost no natural light to come in.

Each room needs to be furnished in different styles and decorated with curtains or draperies of appropriate color and size. Your task is to make the appearance of the rooms as pleasing and elegant as possible.

The task must be accomplished within a tight budget and a specified time period. You are expected to work within these constraints. You will be held responsible for completion of the project as specified in a contract and will be judged and rewarded on your ability to complete the assigned task.

You have the freedom to use your experience, judgment, creativity, imagination, and knowledge to get the job done. Since there are already some residents living in a portion of the mansion as well as the adjoining house, you are expected to finish the project with a minimum of inconvenience and disruption to these folks while the renovation work is in progress.

Now you are on your own. Go ahead and complete the project within the allotted budget and timeline.

Undoubtedly, a tall order, indeed!

The moral of this parable is that for each and every one of us, the need for finding appropriate solutions to many vexing problems is a constant challenge throughout life. There is really no alternative but to gear oneself up and try to find satisfactory solutions to resolve them.

Read on. You will find here plenty of hints, ideas, guidelines, suggestions, case studies and anecdotes lending you a helpful hand in this endeavor. They are instructive, educational, inspirational and, I hope, even entertaining at times!

'It Fits Like a Glove'

Here is a simple example to illustrate this point: To deal with any disease, the prescribed remedy should not create undesirable side-effects which could turn out to be worse than the prevailing ailment. This maxim may be thought of as 'The Principle of Good Fit.' To explain:

Almost everyone is familiar with the saying 'It fits like a glove.' Obviously, a glove should wrap around one's fingers, without feeling too loose or tight—but 'just right.' In the context of decision-making, this principle can best be illustrated with the following diagrams.

Figure 2

A (Circle inside the Square)   B (Square inside a Circle)

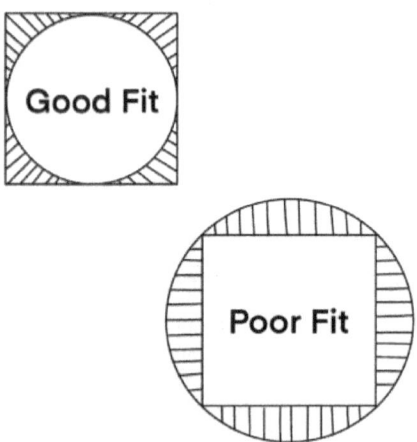

As you can see, the area between the Circle and the Square in Diagram A is smaller than the corresponding area in Diagram B. In Diagram

A, visualize the Square as a 'problem' and the Circle as a 'solution.' In Diagram B, imagine the Circle as the problem and the Square as the solution. Obviously, Diagram A represents a better fit (less wasted space as shown by the shaded area). The Circle in Diagram A hugs the Square much better than the Square does inside the Circle in Diagram B. In other words, the wasted space in A is only about 20% compared to 33% in B.

Whenever and wherever possible, decision-makers should pay attention to the 'goodness of fit' between a problem and its solution. This means that there are no hidden costs or negative externalities which can come to haunt you later, after the decision is implemented.

Chapter II

The Basic Building Blocks

We continue our journey of the decision-making process by introducing some basic concepts and terminology. Regardless of the types of decisions (simple or complex, urgent or non-urgent, short-term or long-term), it is best to start the process by asking a few pertinent questions.

First, the Essential W's:

1. **What** do I want to accomplish? Is this important to my future wellbeing? What kinds of benefits can I expect if I carry it out? What are the associated costs? What is the 'timeframe' for its expected completion?

2. **Why** should this task be done at this period of time? If not, what will happen, and what consequences will follow?

3. **When** should this decision be made? Is it urgent, or can it wait for a while? Will this task occupy a great deal of time, and if so, can it be done in stages?

4. **Where** is the action going to take place? Is it to be accomplished at home, or elsewhere? Near or far? Does it involve travel? If so, when?

5. **Who**, besides myself, should have input and responsibility for this decision and for its implementation? Should others (outside the family members) be included or involved? Can this task be assigned

(delegated) to somebody else? If this is a 'team effort' or a joint decision, is everyone aware of their respective assignments?

6. **How** will this project be carried out? Is there a clear, step-by-step, well-designed plan of action for its execution? Are there any ambiguities in this plan?

7. **Whom** will this decision ultimately benefit, aside from the decision-maker(s)? Are all the potential beneficiaries (outsiders) clearly identified?

Note: This question comes into play when the decision has 'external effects'—as is the case with projects directly/indirectly affecting neighbors/third parties.

To illustrate the importance of these 'W's, here is an admittedly simple, everyday example. It brings out the essential elements of the process. It is the first step in a long journey through the decision-making landscape.

Mark feels hungry. This is the 'trigger point' for the ensuing decision. Distressed by the pangs of hunger, he wants to eat. Now he is ready to carry out a decision. (Note that staying hungry is also an option, which Mark rejects.)

When? If the urge to satisfy his hunger is urgent, it cannot be postponed for a later time. The answer is 'I must eat right now' or as soon as possible. Eating cannot wait beyond a reasonable length of time, perhaps beyond thirty minutes (For some people, hunger can bring about a severe headache or other ailments.)

What should I eat?

This question can sometimes be problematic. Umpteen food choices may be available, depending on circumstances. Sometimes the choices can be baffling, especially if you don't know what you really want.

Have you ever encountered this 'selection problem,' either at a food court or surveying an elaborately prepared 'buffet'? You might have noticed guests walking around, wondering what to put on their plates. Those selections can be numerous and sometimes even confusing—isn't it hard to make up your mind?

In Mark's case, he has definite food preferences. He knows his mind, which makes his choice easy. "Better stick with what I know I will enjoy rather than experiment now" is how Mark solves this problem.

Where should I eat?

If Mark happens to be at home, the menu from which he chooses will probably be limited in scope (and certainly easier). What is readily available in the pantry or the kitchen will dictate his selection. If the food was already prepared earlier, eating can take place almost immediately.

However, since he is away from home, Mark must select a place from the many options that are available. Which one should he pick?

Look at the possibilities. There are several variables to consider. These could range from (a) the quality of food/service expected, (b) the time needed to get food on the table—there could be long waiting lines at the busy lunch hour, to (c) the price.

Besides, there are other factors to consider, depending on one's health/medical condition. Mark is diabetic. There are some restrictions regarding what he can or cannot eat. Which items he can pick depends on (a) freshness of the food being served, (b) its overall nutritional value, (c) calorie content, and (d) suitability to his special situation.

Mark finally spotted some items he liked on the menu. The next question is:

How Much can I afford to spend?

Obviously, the answer depends on his financial wherewithal. Does he want a simple, inexpensive, quick meal? Or perhaps splurge on an especially inviting item that catches his fancy? Does he have a budget in mind?

Mark pulls out his wallet and realizes that he may have to use his credit card, because he does not have enough cash for what he has picked.

How Much should I eat?

This question is not as trivial as it sounds! In Mark's case, because he is diabetic, he must be careful about the quantity (and quality) of food he consumes. The food may taste delicious, but he must restrict the quantity consumed. Otherwise, he knows that his blood sugar levels will spike up. It so happens that the serving size on his plate is more than he wants to, or should, eat. Note that, as a rule, some restaurants tend to serve large portions of food—you can't eat them all right away.

Mark decides to leave a sizeable portion on his plate, to be eaten later. He dislikes wasting food. He had experienced hard times when he was growing up in a poor household. He is reluctant to throw away leftover food.

"Do you want to take a doggie bag home?" asks the friendly and courteous hostess. Mark ponders this question.

Mark now faces a conflict, which must be resolved. Despite his strong preference for conserving food, he is unsure whether it is a good idea to take the 'doggie bag' to his office, where he is headed.

He wonders whether the food might get spoiled before he reaches home later in the evening.

"Yes, thank you. Please pack," he responds. He has momentarily found a solution: he will put the food in the office refrigerator.

Before getting up, Mark must decide one more thing: Depending on his overall satisfaction with the dining experience, he habitually leaves a tip. He wonders how much is appropriate now. He puts a few bucks on the table before heading to the office with the 'doggie bag.'

This somewhat artificial, simplistic and everyday example illustrates many of the W's encountered in making decisions. It sets the stage for exploring other aspects of this fascinating subject. We now turn our attention to this task.

What Decision-makers Bring to the Task

Every decision is made with the aim of moving away from a given status quo to another, more desirable state. People desirous of improving their wellbeing or seeking a better quality of life must be ready and willing to take the steps necessary to reach their cherished goals. This requires motivation, effort, and resources. The mental make-up of the decision-maker at the time of making the decision is critical to its eventual success. Decisions made with a calm, relaxed state of mind and less driven by purely emotional considerations are likely to be more effective. The values you hold that inform the decision as well as the confidence and enthusiasm with which you make the decision are also factors that influence its eventual outcome. The driving force behind many decisions is one's existing philosophy of life and belief system—which encompasses religious, moral, ethical, political, and other socioeconomic dogmas (or doctrines) that you subscribe to and hold dear. They influence your behavior, holding sway over your decisions, working silently and invisibly in the background. They could be encouraging and facilitating those actions or constraining your freedom to act in certain ways. Existing beliefs and habits—which have become part of your personality/ lifestyle—may permit you to do certain things with great ease while only allowing you to do some other things rather gingerly. This is one of the reasons why some people might shy away from certain types of decisions that challenge their traditions or depart from accepted norms of behavior, while others eagerly embrace them.

Anchors:

If you have visited a seaport, you may have observed ships tied (moored) to their 'anchors'—massive, immobile, canon-shaped structures—to hold the vessels in place and prevent them from swaying or moving away. This arrangement (called anchoring) facilitates the smooth and orderly loading and unloading of passengers and cargo.

Likewise, there are certain social/psychological anchors—personal values, philosophy of life, beliefs, and cultural norms—which people adhere to, regardless of where they live and work.

(a) Your Values

Such norms may have evolved over a long period, through the inter-action of various political, social and cultural traditions, giving rise to a common heritage—a 'shared identity.' People living in a certain geo-graphical area may bond together as a distinct entity—calling them-selves a separate nation, ethnic group, or some distinct, identifiable group. A common history or shared experiences also knit them together as a cohesive unit. These factors often give rise to certain well-established 'value systems' or traditions, serving as anchors to guide individual be-havior. Thus, your decisions and choices are partly conditioned by: (a) which society you happen to be part of, (b) where you live and (c) the belief system you have come to accept as the norm.

Various religious, moral, ethical principles and dogmas also exert powerful influence on your outlook and actions. They may permit or prohibit certain types of individual behavior.

Thus, an individual's decisions are not devoid of social context. Rather, strongly held beliefs, whether true or false, right or wrong, shape one's thinking, behavior, and choices. Once certain beliefs take hold, they can limit one's freedom of action. As often happens, they can also stand in the way of rational decision-making by preventing objectivity.

The irony is that while some people swear by their beliefs and defend them fiercely, others may think of them as absurd or meaningless. At the same time, those critics hold on to their own favorite beliefs, which the former group finds equally groundless. Many of these beliefs may have no scientific or rational basis. Indeed, throughout history, many previously popular and widely held beliefs have been proved false, invalid, and meaningless. Despite such evidence, strong believers are reluctant or unwilling to abandon their favorite (false) beliefs. They persist in their convictions, no matter what others think.

Another variant of this phenomenon is popularly referred to as 'superstitions.' Herein you will find the validity of the saying "One man's meat is another's poison." As readers can appreciate, superstitions can either encourage or discourage certain types of decisions. To varying degrees, many people find comfort in their superstitious beliefs, even when they don't help 'good' decision-making. Paradoxically, many superstitions prevent people from making rational choices, as will be discussed in Chapter V.

b) **Resources:**

Making decisions and implementing them requires different types of inputs—collectively known as 'resources.'

For brevity, they can be classified into four categories:

Time, Money, Energy and Skills

These resources are used in varying combinations to carry out activities of daily living. Time is essentially scarce, or limited in quantity, and therefore must be judiciously allocated.

TIME is usually measured in hours, days, weeks, months and/or years:

24 hours per day/365 days per year
4 weeks per month/12 months per year

How one spends (allocates) time among different activities ultimately determines the overall quality of life. This allocation scheme involves:

I.   Studying (Learning, Acquisition of Skills)
II. Working (Earning Money/Purchasing Power)
III. Leisure (Recreation, Sleep, Social/Family Obligations)

Discussion:

#1: Typically, young adults (students) devote the greater part of a day to study and learn. In addition, depending on what educational programs they choose to pursue, the first quarter of life (up to 25 years) may be earmarked for acquiring the various skills necessary to prepare for a chosen career/profession.

#2: Most working parents (adults) typically spend 8 to 10 hours daily for 'work-related/income-generating' activities. Each person must decide how much time should be allocated to work, depending on their preference for income versus leisure.

#3. Dividing one's lifetime among these three major activities—learning, earning and leisure (a generic term for all other activities)—is often dictated by a multitude of factors specific to each person/family. This allocation decision is the primary determinant of one's overall 'quality of life' or personal 'wellbeing.'

In general, most adults typically devote forty to fifty years to 'earning,' i.e., starting from age 20-25 to age 65-70—roughly 2/3 of the average lifespan. The actual number of working years depends on the 'necessity' for lifetime income versus other non-monetary aspects of living.

Learning: 25%;
Working /(Earning): 60%;
Rest of Life: 15%

In general, the first twenty to twenty-five years of life may be devoted to learning; the next forty to fifty years are dedicated to earning money, and the remaining years—the so-called 'Golden Years'—usually entail the retirement phase of life.

However, these phases of life are not mutually exclusive, because:

I.   One can work/earn while learning (as many students do).
II. Learn while earning (lifelong learners or those upgrading skills/qualifications)

III. Continue both learning and earning during the 'Golden' retirement phase.

For purposes of initial decision-making, we must keep these categories separate, to sort out the major issues.

Figure 3: VENN Diagram

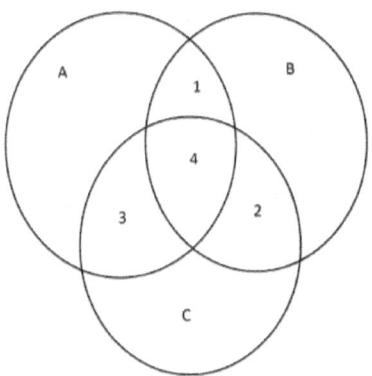

A: Learning   B: Earning / Working   C: Retired

Intersecting Areas: 1 + 4 = Learning + Earning
2 + 4 = Retired and Earning
3 + 4 = Retired and Learning
4 = Retired, Learning and Earning

Discussion:
(1) Students may decide to work part-time while attending school, to finance their education, or may need to supplement their family income.

(2) Working people may need to enroll in courses of study to upgrade their skills.

(3) Retired people may decide to go back to school to learn (for fun) or engage in part-time work to supplement their retirement income.

Figure 4: Typical Lifetime Income Stream

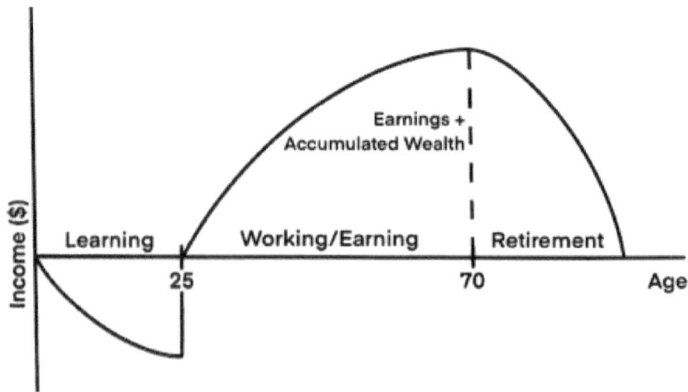

Your lifetime earning power usually depends on the length of schooling as well as the field of specialization chosen. The greater the number of years devoted to learning, the greater is the subsequent lifetime earning power.

One of the most important decisions a young adult must make involves:

(a) What kind of learning/training/preparation for the 'world-of-work' do I need? This question implies that most of us must find a source of lifetime income (usually wage income generated from work) to carry us through.

b) How many years should be devoted to such learning to become reasonably proficient for the chosen field of work? This depends on your income aspirations, based on what work you choose to do, and how much it pays.

c) How much would this learning (education) cost? How can I finance this expenditure? What are the pros and cons of borrowing money for this purpose—constraints versus opportunities?

NOTE: As will be discussed later, one needs to analyze this issue carefully with the tools and techniques of cost-benefit analysis (Chapter IV).

This is a complex, inter-connected and inter-dependent decision.

The complexity stems from several factors, viz: (1) the individual's family circumstances, (2) professional/academic interests of the young adult, (3) financial constraints, and (4) constantly shifting nature of technological change and the work environment.

Discussion:

The level and type of learning one acquires will determine your future earning potential (lifetime income). The appropriate level of professional training should reflect the student's innate academic interests as well as its potential for charting one's future career path, employment opportunities and salary levels. These are unpredictable with any degree of certainty. However, a great deal of useful information and statistics, published by the U.S. Department of Labor and USA/Facts can be consulted to help make an informed decision.

Failure to carry out this important exercise can result in your being saddled with a big 'student debt burden' later in life.

We now resume our discussion of resources.

Money is the financial component of the resource bundle. Some decisions require at least some use of money, either up front or subsubsequently, while carrying out the decision. Several decisions require expenditure of considerable amounts of money, which can act as a critical constraint. These issues are explored in the following pages.

Although the initial endowment of money one possesses (in the resource bundle) may be limited, the underlying goal of many decisions is to increase its future availability. This is especially true of educational and investment decisions. When those decisions are successfully implemented, more income flows can be generated, which in turn become available to enhance wealth creation. Indeed, most of us spend the greater part of our lives pondering questions about money in general—earning, spending, saving, investing, buying, and selling assets and building wealth.

The third component of the resource bundle is **energy**. This consists of four different types:

Physical (muscle) power
Intellectual (analytical/cognitive) abilities
Psychic/Emotional energy
Spiritual energy

Discussion:

Energy, in one form or another, is required to solve most human problems.

Thinking about emerging issues and life's challenges as they arise and finding appropriate solutions for them requires analytical (brain) power.

Carrying out those decisions requires varying amounts of physical, emotional and/or spiritual energy.

Everyday living activities such as walking, climbing, handling utensils, cooking, cleaning, and rearranging furniture, require some physical power. Consider other situations calling for brute physical strength, such as pushing, pulling, lifting, and carrying heavy household items.

Emotional energy is the centerpiece of family dynamics, friendships, and interpersonal relationships. To give and receive emotional support to each other, as and when required, makes it possible for us to cope with the ups and downs of life events.

Spiritual energy is needed to reflect, contemplate, understand, and interpret our unique place in this universe. Humans crave to delve deep into the meaning and purpose of existence—our relationship with Nature and the world around us. Our perpetual quest for peace of mind, happiness and a fulfilling life are integral parts of spiritual energy.

The Fourth component of the resource bundle is your **Skills Set**.

The broadest definition of **skills** is the 'ability to solve problems.' To find solutions to problems is the purpose of making decisions. The set of skills one possesses—both natural (endowed by Nature) and acquired—through formal education, training, work experience, and learning-by-doing—helps us to navigate the ship of life.

Think of your **skills** helping to grow a 'fruit tree', which can produce bountiful harvests for many years to come. Your goal is to nurture and protect this tree so that it can continue to deliver bountiful baskets of sweet, delicious, wholesome fruits to provide nourishment for you and your family.

Constraints

Our freedom to make decisions as well as the ability to execute them effectively is often limited by multiple constraints. Such constraints are an inescapable fact of life. While some constraints can be overcome with hard work and imaginative solutions, others will remain stubborn, challenging our creativity. The major constraints we encounter in making decisions can be classified as:

(a) Institutional   (c) Technological

(b) Value-based   (d) Resource limitations.

a) **Institutional/Social Constraints:**
   Most of us gladly welcome and accept the various social, legal, and ethical constraints that limit our freedom of action, because they are essential for the smooth functioning of a civilized society. Without them, anarchy would prevail.

b) **Value Constraints or Self-Imposed Limitations:**
   Family obligations, professional responsibilities, and adherence to certain personal codes of conduct—are integral to a happy and fulfilling life. Indeed, they provide the rationale (bedrock anchors) to everything we choose to do.

c) **Technological Constraints** are based on what is feasible and practical at any given time, given the existing state of knowledge in any given field.

d) **Resource Limitations:**

The paucity of resources in general—time, money, energy and skills—gives rise to scarcity. Our (material) needs, wants, desires and wishes are almost limitless. No one can satisfy them all. Therefore, one must learn to economize and try to make the best possible use of available resources. Judicious resource allocation helps you to get the 'most bang for the buck.' This means making intelligent, practical, and sensible choices—the theme of this book!

The greater part of what follows in this section is devoted to studying how this can be done.

First, look at **time**.

There are just 24 hours in each day. You cannot do everything you may want to do within that time span. At least this is the common experience for most of us. Therefore, one must pick and choose; some tasks will get done, while others must be left out. This naturally takes us to the concept of prioritizing—the art of knowing how to select what is essential and truly important.

Money: Our ability to spend is constrained by our income (and possibly savings or current assets). Indeed, most readers are familiar with this constraint. How do you choose among the hundreds of goods and services you would like to have? Which need, want, or desire should be satisfied first, and which ones should be left out? Or postponed for another time? We must work within a budget constraint. This means you must 'order' your priorities carefully and make choices among competing uses of available funds.

This principle applies to all forms of **Energy**—the third category of resource. Surely, our physical, intellectual, emotional/psychic, and spiritual energies must be divided and apportioned among competing tasks in a responsible manner. Otherwise, you will feel stressed out, overworked, emotionally drained, and unable to function effectively. Everyone must design a viable strategy to put their energies to good use and purposefully conserve them for the future.

Likewise, the quantity and quality of the skills you possess (whether natural or acquired) act as constraints during different stages of the lifecycle. Fortunately, some of those limitations can be overcome by making smart choices—as explained in the chapter on **outsourcing.**

The foregoing discussion naturally leads to a discussion of:

e) **Priorities**

Since the limitation of resources acts as a powerful constraint on our freedom of action, one must resort to a meaningful selection process—called 'prioritizing.' This means deciding which one of the many competing claims on resources should be assigned the highest 'value' (satisfaction index). A hierarchy of wants should be established, in decreasing order of importance, depending on your tastes and preferences at any given time.

Simple as it may appear, the key to prioritizing is to "know thyself." Only you can know what your innermost values, tastes and preferences are. It is up to you to review them carefully and then pick and choose what is truly important, leaving aside others for later consideration.

To clarify this point, let me illustrate with a real-life example.

People who live in adjacent residential areas (identified by zip codes), also known as subdivisions, usually have similar incomes and may belong to the same socioeconomic class.

"Birds of the same feather gather together" is one way to describe this phenomenon. How they spend their incomes depends on what they consider most important, reflecting their preferred lifestyles. The following five families, almost similar in age, educational and professional backgrounds, choose to spend their money in vastly different ways. Their priorities dictate these choices:

1. The JONES family sends their youngsters to private schools and their college-bound kids to Ivy League institutions, costing a hundred thousand dollars per year.

2. The KING family goes on exotic European vacations or takes luxurious world-class cruises every year.

3. Without blinking an eye, the LARSENS spend money lavishly on frequent dinners in exclusive restaurants, sports and cultural events, Broadway plays, museums, and participate in golf/tennis tournaments.

4. The MONROE household is reputed to have exquisite tastes in antique furniture, paintings, and decorations—so much so that their home has the appearance of a beautiful art museum—which is the envy of the entire neighborhood.

5. Everyone notices that the NORTONS have three new, shiny, expensive, 'prestige' model automobiles parked on their driveway. They seem to be able to trade in their three-year- old models frequently without 'blinking an eye,' as some neighbors put it.

"How do they do it? How come we can't live like them? What is their secret?" is the constant refrain (gossip) around them.

The answers are intriguing as well as instructive.

Each one of these five families choose to spend their incomes in ways that give them the greatest pleasure and satisfaction. Their vastly different lifestyles reflect their values and priorities.

Here is their secret:

(a) The JONES family wants to provide what they believe to be the highest-quality education for their children. They don't much care about cars, exotic vacations or entertaining. They prefer a simple, laid-back, almost frugal lifestyle and live accordingly, to provide for their children's educational needs. They had single-mindedly saved up money for this purpose over many years.

(b) The KINGS enjoy traveling and seeing the world. They decided, long ago, to give up the outwardly luxurious lifestyle of some of their neighbors. To satisfy their hunger for sightseeing and adventure, and to learn about other cultures and peoples, they are clinging to their nomadic way of life.

(c) No doubt the LARSENS send their kids to the local community college and have no appetite for travel or exotic automobiles. They are satisfied with their easygoing, 'enjoy life today' philosophy, reflecting their hedonistic outlook.

(d) As for the MONROES, they really enjoy living in their beautifully appointed 'castle.' They concur with: 'Your home is your castle' approach to life. They delight in 'showing off' their exquisite tastes in art, antiques, and furniture. To them, other types of spending, preferred by their neighbors, do not provide any appeal.

(e) You guessed it: Some may think of the NORTONS as 'car crazy'—but they truly enjoy driving those latest-model vehicles and devote a great deal of time to take care of them as well—washing, waxing and polishing their cars frequently, almost 'babying' them! Their idea of the good life is to buy, drive and trade fashionable automobiles as often as they can. They are avid readers of magazines such as Racing, Motor Trend, Car & Driver, etc. Other forms of spending money—lavish parties, sports, entertainment, travel, clothing and jewelry, etc.—do not interest them.

The Takeaway from this discussion:

Notice that each family has its priorities figured out carefully.

When allocating scarce resources, each one of them has pondered these questions:

"What do I really want? How important is it to me? What am I willing to give up so that I can get my most favorite/desirable things?"

Each of these families has answered this question to their satisfaction.

A well-known proverb sums it all up:

"You can have some of the things all of the time; many of the things some of the time; but not everything all of the time."

Appearances to the contrary, no family, however outwardly rich it may seem, can afford to indulge in every whim or fancy they dream about. Each family has learnt to prioritize and use their resources as they see fit. These families have figured out what they really want and remain satisfied with their choices. They concentrate their energies in doing what befits their chosen lifestyles.

(f) **Beliefs and Habits**

Role of beliefs and habits in making decisions:

Most of us hold certain beliefs that are dear and important to us. By its very nature, a belief system is based on certain assumptions or conjectures about the world, states of nature, social relationships, and lifetime experiences of generations gone by. They also reflect the prevailing structure of the society in which you are born and brought up. Beliefs could be true or false from a scientific point of view. Beliefs that are well established, widely accepted and willingly followed by a certain group of people may look strange, even meaningless, to others who live in another culture or geographical area. Once a belief system gets established and adopted, most adherents accept them without question. They serve as anchors, providing the rationale for legal decisions and actions. Religious doctrines as well as political, economic, social, and legal customs and institutions in every society are built around an underlying belief system. It continues to remain stable until it is discarded, overthrown, or replaced by another belief system. This is an evolutionary process and has happened throughout history—and continues to shape events in our own day.

In some autocratic and tradition-bound cultures, individuals who do not subscribe to or follow the prevailing belief system may be ostracized or punished. Dissidents who question or fail to observe certain customs or beliefs may be shunned, publicly shamed, and forced to conform. Severe penalties may be imposed on them. Under such circumstances, it becomes difficult for those individuals to make decisions that presume to challenge accepted norms and practices. They may either decide to suffer in silence or move elsewhere to escape persecution. That is why the Pilgrims, facing religious persecution, decided to sail to America on the Mayflower and establish their new colony in Plymouth in 1643.

Any belief system, old or new, which stands in the way of making rational decisions should be carefully examined or modified.

Ask yourself:

1. Is adherence to this belief preventing me from making sound, smart decisions that will promote my future well-being and enhance the quality of life?

2. Is this belief constraining my freedom to act logically and rationally?

3. Does this belief make any sense in today's world? Does it have any validity, regardless of when and where it originated? How can I justify holding on to it?

4. How is this belief going to influence my future if I continue to hold on to it? Does it have any intrinsic merit?

5. What will happen if I choose to discard it?

6. Am I being held prisoner (hostage) by subscribing to this belief in any way?

7. Will the benefit of discarding this belief provide me with sufficient compensation for the consequent discomfort/pain/negative impact I might experience?

8. Am I holding on to useless superstitions and fallacious beliefs that prevent me from achieving my full potential?

Fortunately, in most modern, Western, democratic societies, people have the freedom to dissent, think for themselves, make decisions and act according to their own convictions. When you find that some widely held beliefs are misguided, self-serving, meaningless, irrational, and exploitative, you are free to dissent, challenge and reject them. One's decisions ought to be based on knowledge-based facts, not the questionable opinions and superstitious beliefs of ages gone by.

How Habits Can Help, Hurt or Abort Your Decisions

Regardless of whether you realize their presence or not, habits hold considerable sway over how we live and what we do every day. They are silently working incognito, unnoticed and obscure, yet exercising their power and influence over your decisions! Many of your habits were developed and cultivated over long periods of time, consciously or unconsciously, through repeated practice. While some habits take root quickly, others must be carefully nurtured and practiced before they become well entrenched. Once a habit is formed, it attaches itself to your personality like an adhesive or glue, becoming an integral part of your life. They can become addictive and must be attended to (or satisfied), or they will relentlessly nag you to no end, like a hungry infant who must be fed when it starts crying.

Your habits do not care whether they are called 'good' or 'bad,' right or wrong, helpful or hurtful, positive or negative, master or servant. They simply exist because you brought them into existence. You created them; they are just like your progeny. As such, you are responsible for what they do, how they treat you and how they eventually shape your life.

I like to classify habits into two categories—depending on whether they help or hinder your decisions. Those that help to carry out your decisions, promoting your wellbeing and assisting you to reach your goals, can be considered as loyal employees because they serve your best interests as dutiful assistants do. On the other hand, those habits that strangle your self-control, relentlessly gnawing at your willpower and preventing you from carrying out your decisions, are like willful, tyrannical masters (bosses) who only care about themselves! They just sap your energy.

How can this be?

Here are a few examples.

People who want to free themselves from the clutches of 'bad habits'—and decide to improve their lives—must first overcome 'addictive' behaviors which have imperiled their health and wellbeing.

1. The burden of crushing debt.

Despite repeated refinancing of old accumulated debt and participation in mandatory credit counseling sessions, many shopaholics are unable to control their spending habits. They cannot resist the urge to shop, hunting for bargains. "After all, it is Christmas; it comes only once a year; I deserve a break from the tedium of a hermit's life" provides the rationale to splurge, piling on new credit card purchases on top of what is already an excessive debt burden.

One's willpower to control spending melts down like snow on a warm, sunny winter day. Before you know it, monthly payments on the new credit card bills begin to pile up relentlessly, wiping out the benefits of carefully structured debt-repayment plans. You are back in the old rut, monthly bills exceeding income.

2. The opioid epidemic.

At first, those pills provided relief from crushing pain, much needed physical and psychological comfort and improved your ability to function. Gradually you needed much greater doses to provide the same level of relief from pain. Soon you became the victim/slave of ever higher and larger doses of those pain-reducing substances. Their efficacy continued to decline exponentially, as you swallowed greater quantities over time. Like an alcoholic, you now cannot live without them; before you know it, the drug has enslaved you completely.

3. The obesity epidemic

Eating tasty and delicious food is pleasurable, especially when it is sweet, creamy, salty, fatty, and loaded with calories. You get used to taking more and more bites (or sips of that sweet soda) and cannot bring yourself to stop when watching your favorite TV shows or playing video games—which are also temptingly addictive. Those calories stick to your body; you put on weight, gradually becoming obese, and now you want to 'lose weight.' You had spent hundreds of dollars buying unhealthy snacks; now you are prepared to spend hundreds more to lose those unwanted pounds. You want to go on a 'diet' but lack self-control and willpower to start today. You promise yourself: "I will start on my next birthday or on New Year's Day." But that too becomes a pipe dream, forgotten, neglected, unfulfilled and abandoned!

What is to be done to control and get rid of these pernicious habits, which have become tyrannical masters?

There is a remedy:

Remember: "The journey of a thousand miles begins with the first step" — This Chinese Proverb sums it up beautifully!

Here are some suggestions to get you started on the path to free yourself from the clutches of those habits:

1. Determine that you want to fight this psychological war to a successful conclusion.
2. Make up your mind to start today, not later.

3. Knowing the enemy's strength, steel yourself to vanquish them, no matter what it takes.
4. It will take a long time. Prepare yourself for a protracted 'fight to the finish.'
5. Ask yourself:

   When do I want to be debt-free?

   When am I going to be master of my financial life?

   When do I want to get rid of all this high-interest, expensive, crushing debt?

   Or the unwanted, burdensome weight I am adding to my precious body by eating this junk food?

   Or drinking that seductive, poisonous liquid?

   I want to become a happy, self-respecting, disease-free, agile, healthy individual. To do so, I need to change my current lifestyle. If I fail to get rid of these unhealthy, destructive habits, what is going to happen to my body, mind, health, wealth, and wellbeing? Isn't my cherished goal of getting control of these destructive habits worth fighting for, even if it is hard and difficult?

   "Yes: I shall 'tame this wild beast' before it destroys me."

   You are ready to start now.

Go slow, bit by bit. Take your time. So long as you are making progress toward reducing your burdensome debt, losing weight, and reducing the intake of opioids in ever slightly smaller doses, you are on the road to recovery. You are getting ahead. You are gaining control of those habits that had previously enslaved you.

Cultivating Helpful Habits

Many books have been written on the importance of developing 'good and effective habits,' which can propel you toward achieving your goals, become more productive and enhance your quality of life. Here are two worth reading:

Stephen Covey: The 7 Habits of Highly Effective People, Free Press, 1989

Charles Duhigg: The Power of Habits, Random House, 2012

Indeed, there is no dearth of books dispensing good advice on how to improve any aspect of life—for those who want to benefit from reading and practicing those principles and ideas.

The difficulty lies in making them an integral part of your daily life, cultivating and sticking to them until they become daily habits. Thereafter, they will continue to work in the background effortlessly and automatically, helping you to serve your needs.

So, if you want to befriend a desirable habit, you must first feel attracted to it and acknowledge its beneficial potential to enhance your own life. This is no different from "falling in love" or developing a lifelong friendship.

Here is an example:

Suppose you observe somebody cleaning their front yard every day. Their premises are spotlessly clean and attractive. It looks beautiful. You wish you too could do likewise. Gingerly at first, you begin to engage in this somewhat unaccustomed chore. It takes time and effort to do; you gradually get used to doing it, eventually making your own yard look as good as your neighbor's. You may even get complimented for accomplishing the job. You have now acquired a new habit. Hereafter, whenever you fail to attend to this yard-cleaning task, you may feel restless until you get up and start doing it. It now becomes a routine, almost unconscious and even pleasurable. The chore of keeping a clean yard becomes your newly acquired habit, something you may enjoy doing, enhancing the quality of life.

Conclusion: Habits, whether positive or negative, once acquired, become part of who you are. You can choose to nourish those habits you want to cultivate and starve those (negative or harmful ones) you wish to discard. This too is a decision worth pondering.

Reaching Your Goals with Smart Decisions

A 'smart' decision is one that makes use of all available information and then commits oneself to a definite course of action that has a high probability of accomplishing the stated goal.

To accomplish this, the most important criterion is to know what one really wants. Most decisions are based on three fundamental premises or anchors that guide human behavior.

1. You adhere to a given set of 'values' you consider important for your long-term mental/spiritual wellbeing. These 'values' reflect your basic philosophy of life. They set the parameters within which you want to operate.

2. You have a hierarchy of priorities, which reflect your current needs, wants, desires and dreams. The 'order' of priorities does undergo change from time to time, depending on circumstances.

3. You want to uphold certain ethical principles that will guide your behavior and actions.

Need for Adjustments/Compromises

There are occasions when you may have to make some difficult compromises or negotiations to secure your cherished goal. Here is an example:

You want a certain standard of living, which requires a salary of $95,000 (depending on where you choose to live).

You dislike travel or a long commute to work.

You want flexible hours and freedom to work from home.

A benefits package, which includes generous retirement/healthcare/vacations.

Harmonious & stimulating work environment.

Opportunities for conducting research/personal growth.

This 'wish list' of desirable job attributes may be difficult or impossible to achieve. You will have to make some compromises, which require a fundamental reassessment of your current priorities.

What is most important to you in securing an acceptable job?

Can you accept "fixed" working hours in an office environment?

Is (1) a high percent employer contribution to your retirement plan, (2) generous health benefits, or (3) an extended vacation plan more important to you? What is the 'trade-off' among these?

How much inconvenience in terms of 'travel time' are you willing to tolerate/give up for a higher salary?

Or a less desirable residential location?

When you factor in all these attributes (salary, working conditions, residential choices, etc.), you can decide whether the resulting package is acceptable or not.

Quality of Life

The purpose of decision-making is to resolve existing problems that vex us and find solutions to obstacles that stand in the way of achieving a good 'quality of life.' In our quest to seek a better, more satisfying life, we are constantly engaged in efforts to preserve, protect, and improve upon the current status quo whenever possible. Regardless of who you are and where you live, Nature seems to have programmed us to seek and find peace of mind, comfort, and joy in everyday living. This means that all of us are perpetually engaged in seeking whatever we value and want out of life, trying to attain that desirable but often elusive and harmonious equilibrium.

The notion of 'a good quality of life' can be interpreted in many ways. Most readers will probably agree that at a minimum, this includes:

1. Good physical health—the various limbs and bodily organs are performing satisfactorily, as Nature intended them to do.
2. Mental, emotional, and spiritual wellbeing—a tranquil and balanced state of mind.
3. Having loving, rewarding, and satisfying personal/family relationships.
4. A job/career/occupation that provides a dependable and steady stream of income.
5. Adequate leisure time/activities to engage your unique personal interests.

6. Whenever and wherever possible, opportunities to contribute to the 'common good' through purposeful and meaningful activities.

Our journey through life, from cradle to grave, can be compared to a jigsaw puzzle. One tries to organize and put together the various parts of the puzzle and find satisfaction in doing so.

This lifelong enterprise can only be accomplished by making relevant, meaningful, and well-thought-out decisions and carrying them out patiently and diligently. Though often a challenging and intriguing task, the process can be fulfilling in the end.

To achieve one's cherished goals, we must set in motion a blueprint for action and follow it through. The entire process must be supported by adequate resources, a sympathetic personal belief system, helpful habits, and a deep sense of commitment.

What to do:

A. Take stock of the gap that exists between your aspirations (what you truly want to do or achieve) and the current status quo. This helps to assess what needs to be done to bridge that gap.
B. Draw up an Action Plan that will help you to reach your goal.
C. Make an inventory of all the resources needed to carry out the action plan.
D. Visualize the potential challenges, obstacles, difficulties, and problems that you may encounter along the way—in the process of bringing about this transformation.
E. Ask yourself: Am I sincerely willing and able to carry out the action plan, knowing what it entails?
F. Are the potential benefits worth the costs?

G. Is your enthusiasm, determination, and commitment adequate to the task? If so, a decision can be made to move ahead to implement the action plan. Otherwise, pause and reflect.

In the following pages, these questions as well as many others will be addressed systematically, one after another. The author hopes that readers will find them practical and helpful.

Let me start with an example.

Choosing a Career

"I picked my career because I made good money, but I had absolutely no passion for it," says Paul Giannone, who spent thirty years in the field of Information Technology. To many readers, this might seem like a very narrow approach to deciding how to choose a lifelong career.

People pick a career with multiple goals in mind. Probably the most important of these is to derive a steady, dependable income during one's working life. If there are no other independent sources of income—such as an inheritance, royalties, or annuity payment from an endowment—then one must seek suitable employment opportunities to make a living.

In doing so, it is important to bear in mind the distinction between a job, career and profession.

The typical employment ladder starts with an initial job offer—which then leads to many different assignments or positions with increasing levels of responsibility—progressing toward a multi-faceted career, marching toward what may be loosely defined as a profession.

Throughout this journey, you are seeking to derive psychic satisfaction by linking your educational qualifications/talents with available job opportunities for 'professional growth' in a chosen field (of specialization). For many people, "what you do to make a living" is often associated with their personal pride, social identity and status in society. Here is a list of some common attributes most people are looking for in this quest for personal recognition:

1. Adequate financial compensation commensurate with your qualifications
2. Opportunities for promotion/career advancement
3. Stimulating colleagues/challenging work environment
4. A satisfactory package of fringe benefits such as healthcare, retirement income, job security and vacations, etc.
5. Convenient commuting/flexible travel arrangements
6. Availability of affordable housing, educational facilities for children and employment opportunities for spouse (in the case of two-income couples).

In the final analysis, picking a suitable career requires a great deal of soul-searching and compromises. There are many competing and conflicting considerations to deal with. Resolving them satisfactorily and making an informed choice will have a profound impact in enhancing the overall quality of life.

How to Proceed

There is a great deal of similarity among decision situations such as (1) choosing a field of specialization, (2) picking a suitable educational institution to pursue one's educational goals, (3) career choices, (4) residential/

relocation choices, (5) spouse selection, and (6) retirement planning & investment selection. At every stage of life, one is confronted with having to make critical choices with far-reaching consequences impacting the future quality of life. To make the task manageable as well as meaningful, you must devise a system that incorporates your prevailing values, beliefs, attitudes, personality, and personal/family circumstances—and then pick the best option available that fits your specific needs. Your priorities can be reflected in constructing a so-called GRID system by assigning appropriate numerical values to each characteristic you consider important. The numbers you assign to each characteristic are purely subjective, reflecting what matters to you. They range from 0 to 10. Here is an example applied to the job-selection scenario:

Table 2: Grid Showing Different Job Characteristics

	Job A	Job B	Job C
Salary	8	6	4
Work Environment	4	6	3
Level of Responsibility	6	8	7
Commuting	3	4	2
Fringe Benefits Package	7	6	7
Family Considerations	8	6	9
Location	5	4	7
Cost of Living	5	7	4
Total Score	46	47	43

Discussion:

This method can be helpful in those decision situations where there are multiple considerations impacting the final selection. Unless you are willing and able to assign a numerical value to every desirable/undesirable characteristic, it would be hard to come up with a meaningful choice.

Trusting your 'gut' or 'instinct' may work for some people some of the time, but not for everyone. Therefore, the GRID method can be used to supplement/verify/validate what you would have chosen otherwise. It may sometimes help to reinforce your initial impressions/independent judgment.

I must point out that the GRID system has severe limitations. It may not be possible or even desirable to assign numeric weights to situations involving one's emotions, or hard-to-evaluate personality characteristics of another individual. As they say, it must be taken 'with a grain of salt'!

Figure 5: A Four-Legged Stool to Stand Upon

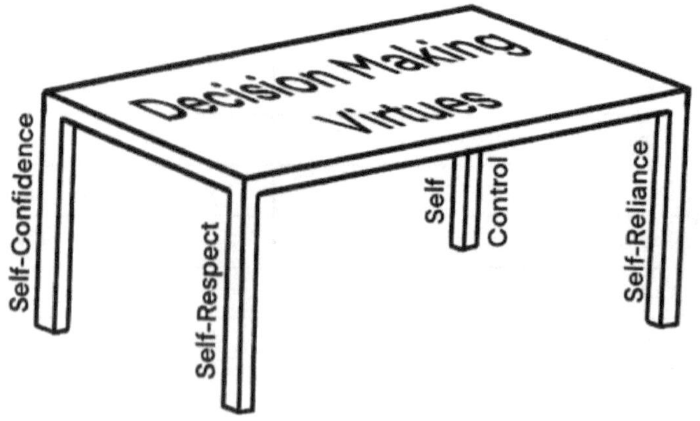

There are four important, worthy, and useful traits that can help the process of making sound, smart decisions: These are: self-respect, self-confidence, self-control, and self-reliance.

Self Respect emanates from a conscious recognition of one's own innate goodness. Having a sense of 'self-worth,' trusting yourself to 'do the right thing' and conducting oneself with dignity are the essential traits of a self-respecting individual. It is the foundation on which one can build a productive and rewarding life. Self-respect is inextricably connected with your Ego. It is born of the realization that one is capable of independent judgment without having to emulate what others say or do. A self-respecting person does not seek constant adulation, praise, or recognition of their accomplishments. However, unsolicited positive feedbacks from others can contribute to building and boosting one's self-respect.

Being true to one's own convictions, regardless of external criticism, is the hallmark of a self-respecting individual. They are not seeking popularity or dependent on approval from others, knowing that their choices are anchored in deeply held moral/ethical values. They are authentic individuals, willing to accept responsibility for their decisions. Shifting blame to others for their mistakes is alien to their nature.

Self Confidence implies readiness, willingness and ability to manage life's challenges in one's unique fashion. Being able to make up your mind to solve emerging problems, plan your future by making appropriate decisions and acting upon them in a timely fashion are important attributes for success in life. These traits come naturally to self-confident individuals. Regardless of what others may think, say or do, such individuals know

71

that it is up to them to conduct themselves according to the dictates of their own conscience. They do not make apologies for their choices, nor do they seek nods of approval from others.

Without confidence in your judgment and readiness to accept the consequences of your actions, one cannot function effectively for long. Self-confidence comes from knowing yourself, your values, strengths, weaknesses, and trusting yourself to be able to live life on your own terms.

Self Control implies complete willingness to admit responsibility for one's decisions regardless of whether they turned out well or otherwise. To paraphrase Ralph Waldo Emerson's words: "I know what I am doing; I have carefully studied the problem; I am confident that the decision I made was the right one and I accept full responsibility for the consequences."

In other words, 'The Buck Stops Here' is their motto, as President Truman was fond of saying.

Self-Control implies a 'measured, thoughtful and studied reaction' to external stimuli. For example, when someone happens to say or do something that makes you upset or angry, most people react in like manner—which usually results in escalating an already tense situation. If, instead, you could assess the situation calmly and sort out what caused the initial furor, your (reflective) response might help to reduce the underlying tension. This requires a great deal of self-control, mental discipline and practice.

Life is replete with situations involving interaction with other fellow human beings whose personalities, attitudes, upbringing, and experiences are vastly different from your own.

Occasionally, some of the people with whom we must interact can be highly irritable, impatient, selfish, or brash. It helps to be civil and cordial toward them, by exercising some degree of self-control to avoid an otherwise unpleasant confrontation. Everyone can thus benefit from keeping 'their cool,' rather than bursting out of control.

Self-control is a great virtue. It does not come naturally to most of us but must be practiced with utmost diligence. The resulting payoff can be priceless. It can prevent many impetuous decisions that often end up causing harm to oneself or others. To the extent that one can gain a modicum of mastery over one's own impulsive actions, self-control paves the way for achieving a better balance between expediency and the common good.

Finally, the 4th leg of the stool is:

Self-Reliance: The self-reliant person goes through life with the conviction that "God helps those who help themselves." This philosophy is the guiding principle behind their decisions and actions. They try to be self-sufficient in the way they live, imposing the least demand on others—society in general—physically, financially, and emotionally. Their motto in life is: 'I will endeavor to take care of myself as best as I can without bothering others.' They try to solve their problems without seeking much outside help—preferring instead to 'make do' with their own (meager) resources. They are proud of their independence, which they try to preserve at all costs.

Self-reliance implies toughness, the ability to deal with hardship and adversity, with as much stoicism as possible. Their motto in life is: "It is better to light a candle rather than to curse the darkness." Rather than complaining about how bad things are, they try to do whatever is within their power to alleviate the distress they see around them. Being self-reliant helps them to live the 'life you want for yourself,' as exemplified by David Thoreau in his celebrated **Walden Pond**.

Conclusion: Those who are endowed with these qualities can deal with the vicissitudes of life with equanimity and grace. Undoubtedly the task of making sound decisions and carrying them out to a successful conclusion can be facilitated by cultivating and nurturing these traits.

These four attributes, while eminently desirable and useful, are neither necessary nor sufficient for making decisions. More to the point, they are indicative of one's character and outlook on life. Those who are endowed with these qualities can deal with the vicissitudes of life much better than others. Undoubtedly, the task of making sound decisions and carrying them out to a successful conclusion is facilitated by cultivating and nurturing these qualities.

Chance vs. Choice

The course of your life is shaped by a combination of two disparate forces: (1) random events outside one's control (purely attributable to chance) and (2) deliberate choices made by you and acted upon—based on personal preferences. At different stages of the lifecycle, one of these forces may predominate over the other. Sometimes what happens through chance may turn out to be good and beneficial—therefore welcome; at other times, chance events may turn out to be detrimental to your wellbeing.

Likewise, your own decisions, the choices you made willingly, can either end up being beneficial, improving your life satisfaction—or the opposite, leaving you dissatisfied and unhappy.

If you are afraid to make choices or altogether dislike and avoid the task of choosing any course of action, your life will still meander forward like a river toward its destination. The river simply doesn't know or care where it is headed, what course it will take, and where it will end. It just flows aimlessly, moving forward relentlessly, until it ends up somewhere—almost always merging up with another body of water.

People who by nature are fatalists and believe that whatever happens to them is 'pre- ordained' are generally willing to let chance play the dominant part in their lives. They attribute various life events that happen to them as the 'Will of God.' They are resigned to the vagaries of Fate, whether it brings them positive or negative outcomes. They are unwilling or unable to chart a self-selected path to determine the course of their lives. This philosophical outlook probably gives them solace, comfort, and peace of mind.

What if I cannot or don't want to make decisions on my own?

While most of us are happy and eager to have the freedom and opportunity to make our own decisions, it so happens that not everyone is inclined to do so at all times. Sometimes people are reluctant to make important decisions (or commitments) for several reasons.

1. They may feel that they do not have sufficient knowledge or expertise to pick the right course of action.
2. They may be afraid of potential adverse consequences. The decision could be inherently risky while their risk-tolerance level is especially low.
3. They could be afraid of criticism from others, being unable to justify why they chose a particular action or provide a convincing rationale for it.
4. Or happy to delegate and have someone else make the decision for them. Occasionally lack of confidence in one's own judgment can trigger extreme anxiety when called upon to make a critical decision.

Or you are simply content to leave the responsibility to an expert or trusted agent of your choice. Indeed, when you are emotionally upset or suffering from extreme mental distress, the last thing you should do is to make important decisions.

Sitting on the Fence

There are umpteen other possible explanations for some people's reluctance or hesitation to commit themselves to a definite course of action. When too many options are on the table, with no clear indication of their respective merits or demerits, confusion abounds. These alternatives could be hard to compare, with no easy way to figure out which one deserves your vote. You are left to wonder what could possibly happen to the one you happened to pick. Fear of failure or criticism about what others might say about your choice is sometimes a strong deterrent to action.

Those with limited experience or lacking self-confidence in their own judgment fall prey to this line of reasoning. The possibility that whatever choice they make may not be the 'best one'—in retrospect—leading to regret and despair—is enough to avoid making any choice whatsoever!

Likewise, procrastinators sometimes try to justify their penchant for inaction. If you are convinced that the information available to you is inadequate or unreliable, you may want to postpone the decision until more data become available. One might even wish that the 'problem' would somehow disappear or go away or hope that divine intervention would come to your rescue!

Self-Starters

People who prefer to take matters into their own hands are ready and willing to make choices that reflect their values, desires, tastes, and preferences. They know what they want, set their goals accordingly and are willing to take calculated risks to move forward. They understand that the final outcome of their choice is almost always influenced by external factors beyond their control (the element of Chance). They figure that the extent to which this is true depends on many factors that are hard to fathom.

The premise of this book is that you can transcend (or at least modify) your destiny—if there is such a thing—by making judicious choices based on well-established principles and techniques. This overarching principle can be summed up as "Though the past cannot be changed, the future is in our power to shape."

The advance of civilization and steadily improving material progress we have witnessed during the past century conclusively demonstrates that human ingenuity and natural forces can be combined in a judicious fashion to improve the overall quality of life. Hans Rosling's book: **Factfulness** (Flatiron, 2015), shows how this has been achieved and made possible by harnessing the power of knowledge, human ingenuity and new technologies. It seems reasonable to assume that your journey through life can be made more enjoyable, productive, and rewarding through careful planning and implementing well-thought-out decisions. In the chapters that follow I attempt to show how this can be done.

Decision-making entails the power and ability to shape the course of your life according to your values, wishes and aspirations. This implies that you make those decisions responsibly and with an understanding of their likely consequences. All such decisions should be based on a realistic assessment of available resources and willingness to deploy them as circumstances warrant. Needless to say, this process is challenging and involves many risks. It calls for deep commitment, a concrete and viable plan of action and the necessary discipline to bring it to fruition.

Having a clear vision of what you need to do to reach your goal is paramount. Knowing your strengths and weaknesses help us to determine what is feasible, doable and what is not. Your values, beliefs and habits must be aligned with your goals. Otherwise, they will stand in the way of making steady, tangible progress.

It would be nice if you could assume that your actions would always produce the desired results. Alas, that is not necessarily true. You can be fairly certain that if you implemented a carefully planned decision with gusto, monitored it carefully and followed it through, it would most probably end up as a winner. On those occasions when you fail to accomplish your goals (due to factors beyond your control), you can still feel satisfied that you did everything in your power to do what was humanly possible. Such setbacks should also provide valuable lessons for future projects—rather than being discouraged by unwelcome failures.

Decisiveness vs. Hesitation

Being decisive can often save resources, provided the decision makes sense—after careful consideration of its merits and demerits.

Putting off important decisions is often counter-productive.

Making up your mind releases scarce resources to do other things because you are now freed from the clutches of having to ruminate on "what to do" about a given problem.

Decisiveness comes from clarity of vision. There is no point in putting off a decision because the problem will keep nagging you until you finally make up your mind.

Unlike procrastinators, decisive individuals make up their minds according to certain established criteria and move on to other matters. They are prepared to fail.

Making Choices

The question is: What can you do to reach your goals or solve the everyday problems you face within the context of the constraints you face in an efficient and economical way? What are the instruments available to achieve this objective?

Most problems we face can be solved in many different ways. The decision-maker needs to think clearly about all the possible alternatives available, from which the best one that fits the problem can be chosen.

Suppose you want to travel to New York—next week. There may be many alternatives to reach your destination, such as air, train, bus, driving your car, sharing a ride with someone, hitchhiking, etc.

Some of these choices are more expensive or time-consuming than others. Some may be more desirable or practical. One needs to calculate the total time spent and all the associated costs of different modes of travel (outlay on airline tickets, bus fare, cost of gasoline, food, tolls, parking, and other incidental expenses).

One of these methods may be more convenient, based on your location and proximity to transportation networks. Such factors need to be carefully considered before making up your mind.

How urgent is the travel mission and how much time is available to fulfil it, is an important consideration.

Which method of travel is the most suitable, efficient, and cost-effective? This depends on who the decision-maker is and which of the resources involved (time, money, or other inputs) is the most valuable (scarce) at a given time.

Everything is relative (or contextual).

We always evaluate our current situation (status, wealth, income, health, job, etc.) from the vantage point of where we are at the moment in relation to some other reference point.

Comparisons are made relative to what we have experienced most recently. Gains and losses are often measured in terms of how they relate to what we have known—not in an 'absolute sense' but compared to some reference point. This is what behavioral economists call the "recency effect." A dollar lost or gained may seem insignificant when compared to a thousand dollars. But if you have only two dollars, then a dollar lost or gained is a big deal: it is 50% of what you had. Pleasure and pain, happiness and sorrow, gains and losses, strength of personal relationships and experiences are all 'relative'—the act of comparison is often the driving force behind most of our behaviors and decisions. Comparative measurements or assessments provide proper perspective to many of your decisions.

All decisions must be carried out within a particular timeframe. This depends on several factors: the type of decision, its urgency, expected target date for completion and nature and characteristics of the task. Once a decision has been made, its execution must follow within those constraints.

Opportunity cost/value of time:

We live in a society where the time available to carry out various decisions is always limited; therefore, time is a valuable or scarce resource. The 'economic value of time' is an important consideration in decision-making. Generally speaking, an hour of time is worth what you could earn if you did 'paid work' during that hour—i.e., your personal wage rate. Since your earning power depends on how much a potential employer is willing to pay to hire you, the 'opportunity cost' of time equals that wage rate. This depends on your level of education, skills, competence, and other characteristics the labor market considers valuable.

Many of our goals can be attained in different ways. There are umpteen paths to reach them. One has to seek them out until all possible available alternatives are explored. Some of these could be much easier, cheaper, less time-consuming and more cost-effective than others. It is up to you to think about all available choices so that you can select the best one that fits your particular needs and circumstances. Unless you spend time and energy in seeking them out, they may be hiding in the background beyond your immediate vision.

Getting adequate information:

To further clarify this important step, it is useful to think of this process as the 'information-gathering stage.' Not only should you explore the many options that are possible and available but gather data about their respective costs. Only then can you make an informed choice about which one of them suits your purpose in all respects. This stage of exploration and data gathering is critical. The cost of gathering the requisite information is part of the equation. They are termed 'search costs'. When you are convinced that the additional or incremental costs of information gathering are about equal to the extra benefits provided by such information, this process should come to a halt.

Search Costs

Here are some general guidelines on how much resources should be expended on 'search costs.'

First: One must clearly distinguish between (a) useful & irrelevant information and (b) pertinent knowledge that can be derived therefrom.

Second: How is this information relevant to making an 'informed decision'? How critical is the availability of information for making this particular decision?

Third: What are the dependable/reliable sources of information that can shed light on this issue?

Fourth: How much expenditure of resources—time, money, energy, and skills—should be devoted to this project?

One should only seek information that is truly relevant, timely, cost-effective, and critical to the mission. As a general rule, this depends on the nature of the topic and your familiarity with the subject. Apart from any cash outlays, the amount of time available to conduct your search and the skill with which you can accomplish this task will determine the ultimate search cost. The wealth of information that is available on the Internet is truly staggering. Therefore, one must be selective and careful in weeding out 'wheat' from 'chaff.'

According to what is called the 'marginal principle,' as long as the extra (or additional) benefit from pursuing an activity is greater than or equal to the associated marginal cost (MB > = MC), one should pursue it.

Applying this rule, how much resources should be devoted (at the margin) to search costs depends on the ultimate value of the information sought. The greater this value, the more beneficial it might be to continue searching for additional information. Here are some examples to clarify this point:

1. Travel costs: airline tickets, resorts/hotel bookings, cruises, car rentals, etc.
2. Big-ticket items such as automobiles, household appliances, computer equipment, and furniture and home renovations.

   Depending on your 'wage rate,' you can calculate and determine how many extra dollars you can 'knock off' the offer price by spending an additional hour of your time and (energy) on search/negotiations.
3. Home mortgages, refinances, home-equity loans, car loans:

   You may be able to save thousands of dollars in interest costs by diligently searching for and finding potential lenders nationwide who can offer the lowest interest rate available for your FICO score. Depending on the type of mortgage, amount borrowed and the term period, even a 0.25% reduction in the interest rate can amount to significantly lower monthly payments.
4. Impact of 'transaction costs and fees' on retirement plan accumulations:

   One of the most cost-effective methods of maximizing the growth of your retirement assets such as 401(k) or IRAs is to find custodians who charge low annual maintenance and investment management fees, which are automatically tacked on and deducted from the Account balances.

Here is an hypothetical example (provided by Vanguard) to show how such fees can eat away the growth of your retirement accumulation.

If you invested $100,000, earning 6% with no fees, you would have about $430,000 in 25 years (thanks to the power of compounding).

If you had to pay a 2% 'management fee' (reducing your net return to 4%), the same $100,000 investment would end up with only $260,000 in 25 years!

This means that the 2% fee wipes out almost 40% off the final account value—its negative impact amounting to $170,000!

This happens because the annual 2% fee is taken directly out of the fund's corpus, leaving a smaller fund balance collecting income. The 2% fee may appear to be small, but its impact becomes significantly larger over time. "Money you lose to costs, can compound (increase exponentially) " the longer the period under consideration.

Lesson: Fees can eat away the growth of your investments.

Conclusion: It may be worth your while to spend some extra time, energy, and money on investigating 'transaction costs' (applicable to any investment decision).

Reliable and timely information is essential for effective decision-making. It is critical to the success of any decision. Making sure that you have all the relevant facts and figures also provides comfort and confidence to the decision-maker.

The type of information needed depends on the nature of the decision/problem/issue you are trying to resolve. Here is a rough outline of how to go about securing what you want:

1. Try to determine, as best as possible, the potential impact of the decision on your future health, financial and emotional wellbeing.
2. For example, major decisions such as education, career choice, home buying, spouse selection and relocation/migration must be made with great care.
    a. Your educational choices will impact your lifetime income potential, financial and career prospects, and future standard of living.
    b. Your housing decisions (whether to rent or buy; locational considerations, whether new/existing property; value-price; down payment; mortgage rates; tax consequences; maintenance expenses and overall affordability.
3. Investigate where the required information is available, its reliability and the time and effort required to acquire it.
4. Find out how much it would cost.

In general, this process is governed by what you are ultimately trying to achieve. Application of the 'marginal principle' should guide the data-gathering efforts. The expected benefit from any additional unit of data collected should be greater than or equal to its cost; when this point is reached, further information gathering becomes counter-productive. Remember: 'Information Overload' is not only confusing, but also wasteful.

Here are some examples:

The college selection process:

Once you have determined what type of educational program/major field of study (concentration) sparks your academic interests, one should investigate which college/university will best fit those aspirations. There should be a proper fit between your educational/social/professional goals and the type of institution you eventually pick. This is supremely important, because a mismatch between your personality and the educational/social atmosphere of the institution you happened to pick can be very detrimental to your future. There are obviously several factors that must be considered:

Strength and reputation of the academic program, relative to your personal background and specific interests

Geographical location of the institution, general ambience, housing facilities; distance from home—i.e., travel time and other related expenses.

Net out-of-pocket costs of the educational program in its entirety.

According to the College Board (Trends in College Pricing, 2019), the dropout rate of College enrollees as well as those who failed to complete their degree programs was about 40%. A major reason for this dismal outcome is a failure to pick the right academic program/institution—partly the result of a mismatch between the student and the college, resulting from inadequate data gathering/analysis by prospective candidates.

Indeed, such a cavalier attitude, often mixed with reluctance/unwillingness to invest in adequate information gathering prior to making the educational decision, can ruin your life. Low-income prospects, high unemployment rates and dissatisfaction with life in general can ensue as a result.

Word-of-mouth recommendations, though valuable, do not serve as adequate substitutes for fact-checking and data gathering when it comes to making decisions about healthcare, educational investments, home buying and other critical ventures. Indeed, resources expended in ensuring that you have all the facts and figures relevant to making informed decisions is justified. 'Full disclosure' by all the parties involved must be the rule, not the exception.

Comparing Benefits and Costs:

The next stage of this exercise is to compare all the benefits of the proposed action in relation to its associated costs. One should assess all the potential benefits (monetary, psychic, inter-personal, social) of the selected option. Likewise, all its potential costs should be listed. Then the benefits can be compared with the costs. If the benefits exceed or equal the costs, you can implement the decision; otherwise, no action should be taken.

These general principles are easier stated than followed. One of the most difficult tasks facing the decision-maker is to identify, measure, calculate and delineate all the expected benefits and costs and setting them up side by side. Since there are many possible solutions to a problem, clearly identifying their relative benefits and costs is, at best, a daunting task. However difficult and time-consuming this task may be, a satisfying decision cannot be made unless it is taken seriously and completed. Indeed, failure to do this is one of the main reasons why you may find it difficult to make good (satisfying) decisions.

Good decisions take time to implement. What makes a decision 'good' is precisely the homework done prior to its adoption as the best available option. This requires a lot of hard work, patience, and determination. A dedicated student who is willing and able to spend time and energy doing the requisite homework or research will pass the examination with flying colors. Those who are unwilling or unable to do so cannot perform satisfactorily. Similarly, the decision-maker must do the necessary homework if the decision is going to turn out the way you want and expect. Otherwise, disappointment and regret are bound to follow.

Sometimes your personal decisions may confer various benefits and costs on others. These are called **Externalities**. Although most personal decisions have limited externalities, they do sometimes happen, albeit unintentionally. A good decision-maker must take such externalities into account by weighing them according to their relative importance. For example, my decision to start or quit smoking does confer secondary health costs on others. My decision to inoculate against communicable diseases will have a beneficial external impact on those I come into contact.

Although most people usually ignore such niceties in making their personal decisions, it may be desirable to bear them in mind (to the extent possible), especially when society at large is impacted by your actions.

We will be dealing with this topic in Chapter IV.

Chapter III

The Triggering Mechanisms

Decisions are motivated by a strong desire to achieve some specific goal. The eminent psychologist Abraham Maslow theorized around 1943 that there exists a certain hierarchy of unmet needs that act as a triggering mechanism, inducing people to take action to satisfy them. Maslow argued that these needs can be depicted in a certain order of priorities. They start from the most basic (physiological) needs to progressively loftier ones, which he termed as esteem/self-fulfillment needs (aspirations). Maslow's hierarchical depiction is shaped like a pyramid, made up of five parts, as shown below.

Figure 6: Maslow's Triangle

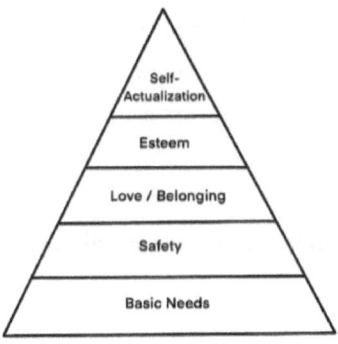

This five-stage model was divided into so-called 'deficiency needs,' which are the bottom four, and 'growth needs,' the 5th (on top).

Maslow's rationale for depicting these needs as a pyramid was that basic physiological needs such as hunger take precedence over safety or emotional needs and then gradually progress toward what he termed 'esteem and self-actualization needs.'

We will take a less structural approach. Decisions may be thought of as attempts designed to solve different problems that vex us, with the ultimate object of improving the overall quality of life. Identifying those problems and methodically seeking and finding feasible solutions to resolve them constitutes the purpose of all decisions. This could be thought of as falling into three distinct categories:

First, to accomplish some new goal such as:

1. Enrollment into a Degree/Certification/Apprenticeship Program to pursue vocational/technical education in a specific field.
2. A college graduate seeking a career in the banking/financial services industry.
3. An entrepreneur applying for a license/permit to start a restaurant/food distribution business.
4. An individual applying for a passport/visa to visit a foreign country to conduct research/study/travel.
5. A couple getting married and/or starting a family.
6. Build/buy a house or acquire rental property.
7. Volunteer in a project to teach disadvantaged/handicapped persons.

8. Conduct scientific research or experiments to study, explore and understand natural phenomena such as earthquakes, hurricanes, tornadoes, etc.

9. Undertake medical research to come up with remedy/treatment for a rare disease.

Second, to seek change from the status-quo, triggered by dissatisfaction with the current situation.

1. Embark on a different career path (moving from teaching high school to an MBA program) with greater challenges/opportunities for professional advancement.

2. Relocate from New York City to another small town in the Midwest to seek a lower tax rate and cut living expenses.

3. Refinance the current mortgage/restructure existing debt to take advantage of lower interest rates.

4. Quit a high-stressed executive position in Stamford and move to a less-hurried, easy-going lifestyle in the Vermont countryside.

5. Sell my house: "I am tired of all the hassle and costs involved in maintaining this property. I want to move to a condo or rental housing before next Spring."

6. Shift investment strategy: "I am dissatisfied with the poor performance of the current stock portfolio. A low-cost-index fund is probably the right way to go at this stage of my life."

Third, take steps to resolve issues/problems that are causing a great deal of **SWAT** (an acronym for Stress, Worry, Anxiety and Tension).

1. "Stress causes, disturbs or interferes with the normal physiological/psychological equilibrium of an organism.

2. Worry is to feel uneasy, fret or torment oneself with disturbing thoughts.

3. Anxiety is a state of mind experiencing distress or uneasiness caused by apprehension of potential danger/misfortune or failure.

4. Tension is equated with mental or emotional strain, especially when one experiences strained relationships/conflicts with individuals or groups".

Although psychologists have provided distinct and varying interpretations of these SWAT terms, it is convenient for us to combine them into an acronym here representing a general state of mental anguish or uneasiness, robbing one's tranquility and peace of mind. Many aspects of our lives are riddled with a plethora of unhappy, unwelcome events, situations and problems, causing a gamut of negative emotional/psychological feelings and physical discomfort. This is a constant, perennial and unwelcome byproduct of our harried lifestyles. As such SWAT, in one form or another, follows us like a shadow everywhere. It not only manages to burden our minds with nagging feelings of inadequacy and inability to effectively manage our lives but diminishes the joy and enjoyment we should experience from living. Often, this manifests itself in the form of a sense of helplessness and lack of personal control. The ultimate effects are pernicious on both our body and mind: i.e. constant irritability, physical exhaustion, sleep deprivation, inability to concentrate and deal with the various tasks on hand that need your attention. Consequently time, energy and money are often wasted in unproductive ways to combat SWAT. Some seek quick relief for their distress in remedies such as drugs, alcohol, smoking, binge eating and compulsive shopping—all of which only compound the problem, jeopardizing their health further, without solving the underlying root causes.

According to a recent report (2021), entitled "Stress in America," published by the American Psychological Association, levels of SWAT experienced by a majority of Americans have increased markedly in the last two years. This could be the result of pandemic-related problems, which have brought about additional strains on working mothers who have to take care of school-age children unable to attend their classes due to Covid-related restrictions. Millions of parents have also lost their jobs, putting their financial lives at risk. In a nutshell, large sections of the population are now facing various types of SWAT-induced chronic physical and mental health problems, compounded by unemployment, inadequate financial resources, and conflict-ridden family dynamics—wondering how to cope and what to do.

Rather than belaboring this point, let us examine how 'smart' decision-making can help to mitigate some of this malaise. There are some things you can do to manage/control SWAT, and some that you cannot. Let us review them.

Ask yourself: Is the SWAT caused by some self-imposed, misguided values and beliefs that have tripped you into doing things and engage in activities that are causing more harm than good?

For example:

1. Lack of time: Many time-starved modern families find themselves always super busy, trying to do too many tasks that cannot all be completed effectively within a certain time period—day,

week or month. Are all these activities really necessary or important?

Do they also make sense? Will these activities/choices help to improve your ultimate quality of life? If the answers to these questions are mostly 'negative'—then you should 'prioritize' some of these tasks. Try to give up what is really not important or contributing to your long-term wellbeing. Concentrate on just a few, and discard others.

Evaluate them carefully and dispassionately. "Don't bite more than you can chew." Or as David Thoreau advised, "Simplify, simplify."

2. Financial strains: Are you spending more than you can afford to? Why are you unable to meet your financial obligations? Finding too many bills in the mailbox? Then look for possible solutions such as:

   (a) Trim your spending as much as possible, right now.

   (b) Consider selling some of your assets (unused jewelry, artwork, other stuff lying around) and use the proceeds to pay off debts carrying high interest rates;

   (c) Try to increase your income temporarily by working overtime or a second job.

   (d) Rearrange (stretch) your monthly payment obligations by investigating and negotiating for cheaper, more affordable loan-terms.

   (e) Find out if someone—family members, friends, employer—can help you out a bit.

   (f) Increase the number of W-4 withholdings temporarily, to increase cash flow (take- home pay).

(g) Reduce your cash outflows—again temporarily—sell a second car, cancel/suspend association-memberships, subscriptions, reduce gifts, donations—as much as you can.

3. Let go and slow down! Trying to win every game, all the time, can take away the real fun. "It is the journey that counts—not the destination"—or 'winning.' Sticking to this wise counsel can save your sanity and free yourself from many unhappy, hopeless situations (such as climbing the proverbial corporate ladder, trying to win every argument, getting ahead of others in sports/competitions, building wealth, and moving forward at a super-fast pace in the 'game of life.'

4. Bend, not break: Trying to change others—their values, habits, beliefs, political and religious affiliations, attitudes, and expectations—generally doesn't work. Other people are just as fastidious as you are. It is far more sensible and productive to change oneself before trying to change others.

5. Practice 'contentment.' Try to enjoy what you have, right now; don't fret over the future too much. Have realistic goals. Keep striving with discipline and determination. Patience and self-control are the twin engines that can contribute to one's physical and mental health.

6. Try generosity: Sharing, caring, and helping those who are less fortunate is a worthy endeavor. Provide physical, emotional, financial, and spiritual comfort to ease the distress and burdens of others—in whichever feasible way you can. This is a great 'stress reliever'; while helping others, you will end up helping yourself as well!

Of course, there are some temporary, ad-hoc, time-honored strategies suggested to cope with SWAT, which are easy to follow:

(1) take a long walk,

(2) listen to music,

(3) smell the flowers,

(4) count your blessings,

(5) read a book such as Dale Carnegie's *How to Stop Worrying and Start Living*

(6) pray, because although "Prayer does not necessarily change things, it changes people and people can change things."

Eisenhower Matrix

One of the factors contributing to high levels of SWAT is a general paucity of time (as well as energy) to attend to and complete the many tasks we encounter every day. General Eisenhower, as Supreme Commander of the Allied Forces, faced this problem. Since it was almost impossible to deal effectively with the multitude of tasks he had to address, Eisenhower devised a strategy to concentrate on some and eschew others, based on the following criteria.

The strategy is designed to prioritize and divide various tasks into two major categories—depending on how "urgent" OR "important" they are. Some of the tasks may be 'urgent'— requiring immediate attention—while others are deemed less 'urgent.' Similarly, some tasks are labelled 'important' because they contribute the 'lion's share' to your achieving your mission (or overall wellbeing), and others are less important. Once the order of 'urgency and importance' are determined, you are able to decide which tasks deserve your immediate attention and which ones can be put on the 'backburner.'

Here is the diagram (matrix) representing division of the tasks, according to the criteria of urgency and importance. The matrix is divided into four squares. The X and Y axes represent 'important' and 'urgent,' respectively. The degree of importance or urgency of a given task can vary from 0 to 100%. Your resources (time, energy, money, etc.) must be allocated among these two distinct and yet competing categories.

Figure 7: Eisenhower Matrix

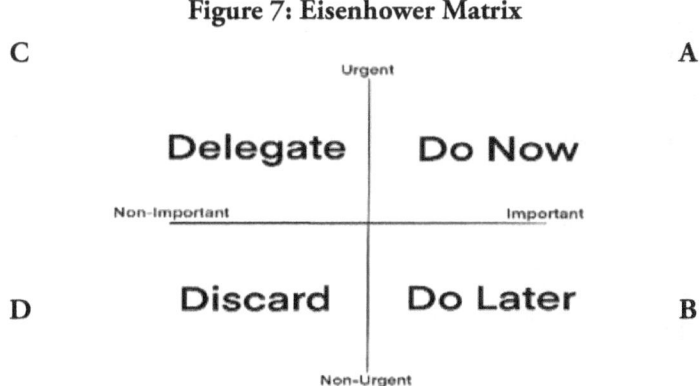

Notice that items that are labelled 'urgent' are not necessarily always 'important'; likewise, some important tasks may or may not be urgent. In certain cases, tasks can be both urgent and important (as in the case of a medical emergency). The level of urgency/importance depends on how soon the task must be completed. (To give an example, a phone call from your boss asking you to attend a meeting scheduled for tomorrow is deemed both U & I.) Failure to comply can have serious consequences. On the other hand, watching your favorite TV show or washing your dirty laundry could be considered urgent, but not important.

Saving for retirement or preparing for a lifelong career are important goals but can be done slowly, over time.

The final draw:

Quadrant A: U & I: Attend to these tasks immediately.

Quadrant B: Important, but not Urgent: Do later, leisurely.

Quadrant C: Urgent, but not Important: Delegate to others.

Quadrant D: Neither Urgent nor Important: Ignore, or discard.

Conclusion:

If you are able to sort out and prioritize all the different tasks, categorize them appropriately and fit into the respective quadrants, you could act upon them as Eisenhower suggests. Then probably a great deal of SWAT could be managed more effectively!

Classification of Decisions

There are many ways to classify decisions: by (1) their frequency of occurrence, (2) types of decisions by subject-matter, (3) degree of ease/difficulty in deciding, (4) urgency or importance, (5) their impact on the overall quality of life and (6) residual or external effects—how it might impact third parties.

Table 3

Types of Decisions

Frequency	Everyday	Now & Then	Infrequent/ Rare
Percentage	80%	15%	5%
Impact on Quality Of Life	Significant	Substantial	Profound
Info. needed	Routine	Moderate	Substantial
Inputs required	Average	Large	Issue dependent
Search Costs	Insignificant	Moderate	Large
Urgency	High	Sometimes	Rarely
Importance	Limited	High	Great
2nd Opinion	No need	Infrequent?	Desirable
Re-consider?	Maybe	Sometimes	Critical

DECISION CHARACTERISTICS

Note: This table arranges decisions according to their major characteristics.

Frequency refers to the sheer number of decisions being made—whether they are repetitive, infrequent, occasional, relatively rare, and so forth—in purely quantitative terms. Using the so-called 80/20 Rule, which applies to many types of phenomena, it appears that a majority of decisions can be classified as frequent—occurring almost on a daily basis—and do not take much time or effort. Roughly 80% of household decisions take up only about 20% of your time. They are mostly 'run of the mill' types of decisions—meaning almost automatic, habitual, even unconscious. You get up in the morning at a certain time, attend to the usual household chores, work, do shopping, engage in family activities, discharge personal obligations, exercise, socialize, entertain, etc.—all done almost automatically or routinely without a great deal of thought or planning. By sheer volume, they probably constitute about 80% of all 'decisions,' while requiring just 20% of time.

The other 20% of decisions require special consideration. They may require a great deal of thinking, planning, critical analysis, and above-average financial outlays. Decisions concerning higher education and fields of study/specialization, charting one's career/professional path, marriage/family formation, residential choices, healthcare, investments, portfolio selection, retirement planning, etc.—require in-depth analysis and reflection because of their potential long-term impact on one's quality of life.

Then there are some decisions which, once made, cannot easily be changed or reversed.

Decisions about marriage/divorce and estate planning/ gifting/ lumpsum distribution vs. periodic payments during the retirement phase of life, belong to this category.

Some decisions, especially those having to do with unexpected events, must be carried out urgently. Emergencies such as sudden illness, accidents, fire, or flood hazards, etc., do not give much time for careful reflection—they must be addressed right away.

As we have seen earlier, a few of these decision-categories are not 'mutually exclusive,' meaning that they could be simultaneously: Urgent & Important; Reversible & Important and so forth.

Certain types of decisions, whether carefully planned or otherwise—can end up having unintended desirable or undesirable impact on third parties—called 'externalities.' This subject is more fully discussed in Chapter IV.

The overriding goal of decision-making, as in many other areas of life, is to solve problems to reduce SWAT, take steps to enhance the overall quality of life and contribute to the wellbeing of society. This often entails costs (sacrifices) in terms of resources—time, energy, money, and skills. The resources available to us are limited in both quantity and quality. Some of your decisions may come to fruition quickly while others may be slow to materialize—the sequence of flows of costs and benefits may be short-lived or last longer, depending on the type of decision.

There are three possible scenarios:

A. Benefits may accrue rapidly (up front); costs to be borne later.
B. Costs must be incurred first, with benefits emerging later.
C. Both costs and benefits flow more or less simultaneously.

Note that the term "flow" implies that both costs and benefits may continue for some period of time, rather than occurring instantaneously.

Smart decision-making involves being conscious of the entire spectrum of costs and benefits, whether they occur 'up front' or emerge slowly later. It is possible that some of these may be clear and obvious, while others could be hiding in the background. All of them must be sorted out and accounted for. Otherwise, the decision is bound to be suboptimal. This state of affairs happens especially when someone other than the 'decision-maker' ends up bearing some of the hidden costs.

In your eagerness to implement a decision whose benefits are quick to materialize (while costs are incurred much later), you may be tempted to act in a hurry. This happens when people decide to indulge in activities such as binge eating, casual sex, smoking, impulse shopping, driving fast zigzagging through congested traffic, talking loudly on cellphones in public places, and discarding plastic bottles outdoors.

In general, when cost outlays precede delayed flow of benefits, there exists a built-in incentive to analyze whether the proposed action is desirable and worthwhile. This is especially true when the upfront monetary outlays are sizeable. Examples are self-financed educational outlays, home buying, relocation and migration, purchase of insurance and annuity contracts.

To summarize, one should be cognizant of the existence of certain hidden or 'implicit costs'—which tend to distort some decisions. When individuals can shift some part of the cost of their decisions to third parties or society at large (taxpayers), there exists a strong incentive to do so. Projects that might not otherwise pass a strict 'cost-benefit test' might then seem temptingly desirable.

It is generally the case that the flow of benefits and costs happen in tandem. This is likely to be true for almost 80% of everyday decisions made by the average American household.

There is another type of decision not discussed so far—philanthropy—which is somewhat unique in the sense it benefits both the giver and the recipient. When people willingly make donations or contributions to help others, "it becomes twice blessed." Those who are on the receiving end can use the money to alleviate their financial distress. The donors may also derive immense psychic satisfaction from the 'act of giving' and knowing that they are able to help the less fortunate sections of society. Willingness to share one's time, talents, knowledge, expertise, money, and other resources—volunteering in the broadest sense—is a laudable decision indeed.

Chapter IV

Some Essential Economic Concepts

Familiarity with certain basic economic concepts is essential for making smart, cost-effective decisions throughout the lifecycle. Most of the questions and issues one must tackle often involve the use of scarce resources. Learning how best to allocate these resources to reach your goals is what economic principles teach us. I provide below a sampling of some of these basic tenets and their applications.

After a brief introduction, several examples and real-life applications are provided to show how everyday decisions make extensive use of these concepts.

I. Opportunity Costs:

There are two basic realities all decision-makers must contend with (in addition to death and taxes!):

1. The resources available under your command are strictly limited.
2. These resources have alternative uses.

What does this mean?

Using a resource in one way makes it unavailable for another use. Therefore, one must be careful about how to allocate it wisely.

This is a dynamic and powerful concept.

Here is why:

Value of Time

When you are working to earn a living, you are 'monetizing' your time (as well as energy—physical, intellectual, etc.) into dollars of 'spending power.' Money commands general purchasing power; therefore, you must convert your time and skills into money to be able to buy the other things you want. The opportunity cost of your time is your wage rate—expressed in terms of $ per hour. This wage rate represents the value of time—what an employer is willing to pay to hire you (per unit of time—hour, day, month, or year).

One of the critical decisions everyone must confront is:

How much time do I want to devote to (or must) work to earn money?

When should I (at what age) do I start working, and when should I quit working? (i.e., retire from the labor force)?

The answers depend on several personal/family circumstances.

Your 'need' for money dictates these choices. Your 'love of work' also enters the picture.

For most of us, earning money is a necessity. The higher the 'wage rate,' the greater are the forces 'pulling' and 'pushing' us in the direction of seeking monetary rewards. People who seek a high material standard of living do choose to work long hours (and years), trading their leisure time for work. This choice is reflected in (a) hours devoted to 'overtime pay,' (b) converting vacation into 'cash,' and (c) taking up a second job or a consulting practice to supplement regular paychecks.

Workaholics naturally enjoy what they do: for them, 'work is worship.'

However, for millions of hourly workers, and most salaried staff, the choice between work and leisure is somewhat problematic. They must contend with the desire for a high material standard of living, vis-a-vis having enough leisure time. Some people work many long hours every day, as well as on weekends. They prefer having more money, no doubt.

Here one may pause and take a deep breath.

1. What do you value most? More $ with less time, or fewer $ with more time? This question is at the heart of many of the debates about "work-life balance"—going on around us.

2. The concept of opportunity cost permeates every aspect of life. Here are some typical situations:

   i) Suppose you have a 'dental emergency' and must spend two hours at the dentist's office. This is an unplanned use of time, which must now displace another previously planned activity.

      Those two hours become unavailable to shop, work, play, sleep, entertain, engage in social activities, etc. One of those activities must be curtailed or given up: this is the opportunity cost of having to undergo emergency dental care.

   (ii) Suppose you have to stay back at your office and work for an extra hour. Now you cannot spend that hour with your family. Consequently, you are deprived of valuable family time.

   (iii)If you are caught in a traffic jam while commuting to work and reach your worksite late, you have unwittingly used up 'work time' (unproductively in this case!). Consequently, some other tasks you had planned to do must be postponed—resulting in financial loss or another lost opportunity.

Such examples abound. When time is literally snatched out of your hands, the resulting 'time deficit' results in mental aggravation and causes stress, anxiety, sleep deprivation and other 'in kind' opportunity costs.

The significance of opportunity costs becomes even more apparent when you consider how one expenditure displaces another. Suppose you are suddenly taken ill and stuck with unexpected medical bills. Your carefully planned budget is now 'bust'! Earlier, you had planned a birthday bash for a loved one. Now you are forced into a difficult choice: either cancel the birthday festivities or borrow money to pay for it. If you decide to borrow, this creates yet another future financial burden: you must come up with funds to pay back the debt—with interest added.

A similar situation exists with respect to current spending vis-a-vis saving for the future. A dollar can be put to umpteen uses today. Once spent, it is gone forever. There is often a 'tug-of-war' going on between current spending and the imperative to save for the future. You rationalize that after paying all those current bills, there is very little money left to save.

Besides, most of us are fixated on the present and too busy to worry about a distant future.

If this pattern of behavior sounds familiar and you are really (seriously) interested in increasing the savings rate, you can 'nudge' yourself to do so. Consider the following:

Present Allocation:

Current spending	98%
Saving	2%

Proposed Allocation:

Spending	90%
Saving	10%

By prioritizing saving and earmarking a larger percentage of income for that purpose, one can decide to raise the saving rate. Rather than treating saving as a 'residual,' you have now decided to elevate it to the first rank!

This will naturally result in reducing the funds available for current spending. Though inconvenient and painful at first, the re-allocation helps you to achieve your savings goal, which was eluding you earlier. As a result, a better balance can be achieved between the present and the future, improving the overall long-term quality of life.

This is the essence of 'opportunity cost,' a 'trade-off' between two competing allocation decisions.

II. Trade-offs

Using a scarce resource in a particular use makes it unavailable for an alternative use. Since wants are unlimited, one must learn how to allocate resources effectively. This is where the concept of 'trade-off' enters the picture. One must decide which 'want' must be satisfied first, thereby sacrificing another one of almost equal value.

Every aspect of living is replete with choices: so, knowing about and willing to accept the associated trade-off is essential to make smart decisions.

Here is an example of a financial calculation to help/decide whether it is worth moving closer to the place of work to save on commuting expenses:

Note: This calculation ignores the following factors:

1. Psychic cost or pleasure experienced by the commuter.
2. The emotional costs of relocating (for the family).
3. Friendships lost/gained in each neighborhood.
4. Non-financial aspects of being closer to work.

Assume the house closer to work costs an extra $50,000—i.e., $300,000 vis-à-vis $250,000 (existing location). Assume that moving saves 25 miles of commute.

1. Costs: Extra monthly mortgage payment on $50,000 at 5% = $208 per month. This will continue for thirty years, for a total cost of $75,000. Can you afford this additional monthly cost? Are you prepared to handle this by making other adjustments in your budget?
2. Benefits: Opportunity cost of time saved by not commuting: Conservative estimate: 1 hour each way: on the commuter train: 20 working days per month: x 2 hours x 12 months: 480 hours @ $50 per hour = roughly $25,000, depending on the average hourly wage of the commuter. Assume that this is the total economic value of commuting hours.

   This continues for thirty years of commuting, meaning a total cost saving of 25,000 x 30 = $750,000.

   Out-of-pocket costs of commuting: $10 a day, assuming a cheap railroad pass.

   Money saved: $10 x 20 days x 12 months x 30 years = $ 72,000.

Conclusion: It is worth moving closer to work. The resulting saving on commuter costs far exceeds the mortgage cost of the house.

Note: These calculations are done in 'present dollars.'

If you were driving to work, a similar calculation would indicate that the saving on gasoline, car maintenance costs/wear-and-tear on the car and the value of driving time saved would justify re-locating closer to work.

III. Comparative Advantage

The underlying logic of the preceding argument applies equally well to other resources—energy and skills. One of the cardinal principles in economics, known as 'comparative advantage,' illustrates this point.

Table 4: Production Chart

	Jack	Jim	Ratios
Nails	60	30	2:1
Hammers	20	5	4:1
Efficiency Ratios	3:1	6:1	

Explanation:

Jack can produce either 60 nails or 20 hammers per day, compared to Jim's 30 nails or 5 hammers. Jack's overall productive superiority is evident in both items. While Jack can produce twice as many nails as Jim, he can turn out four times more hammers. Alternatively, Jack must give up 3 nails to produce 1 hammer, while Jim must forego 6 nails for each hammer. (These ratios are highlighted.)

Although Jack excels in producing both nails and hammers compared with Jim, his comparative advantage (or superiority) lies in the production of hammers (4:1) four-fold, vis-à-vis nail production (2:1).

In other words, Jack's internal (personal) cost is 3 nails for 1 hammer, compared to Jim's internal cost: 6 nails = 1 hammer.

Now, suppose Jack and Jim decide to trade with each other. Jack concentrates on producing just hammers, while Jim takes up making nails exclusively. This new arrangement benefits them both.

Here is why:

Jack agrees to sell one hammer to Jim in exchange for four nails. Jim is only too happy to accept this trade: instead of having to give up (sacrifice) six nails to produce one hammer (which he was doing earlier), he is now better off, having one hammer + two nails after trading with Jack.

How about Jack? He too is better off, getting four nails from Jim for each hammer he sells. When he had to make both items, he could only get three nails per hammer, its 'opportunity cost.'

This mutually beneficial production and trade arrangement resulted from specialization and exchange. Each person decides to concentrate on producing only one item, according to their respective *Comparative Advantages.*

The exchange could also take place at other ratios, such as one hammer = five nails, so long as both agree to do so.

Let us now extend the logic of this argument one step further:

Suppose Jack is good at doing several tasks better than Jim. Each of these tasks require different input of energy/skills. Since Jack is a wizard, he can do everything better, faster, cleaner, nicer, more efficiently, compared to his counterpart, Jim.

Take any six tasks and arrange them in order of descending productivity: A, B, C, D, E and F. If Jack must do everything himself, he feels overwhelmed. If he works six hours, he must spend one hour on each task, frittering away his time, energy, and skills.

Instead, Jack decides to concentrate only on the first three tasks, A, B and C, where his productivity exceeds that of Jim by ten, eight and six times, respectively. His superiority over Jim, in the lower-ranked tasks, D, E and F, is much less—four, three and two.

Likewise, Jim agrees to concentrate exclusively on tasks D, E and F. This new arrangement makes both men better off, instead of each person trying to do everything. Jack hires Jim to do tasks D, E and F, paying him much higher wages—2 or 3-fold (Jack can afford to do this easily, thanks to his superior productivity). Recall that Jim was earlier dissipating his energy on doing tasks A, B, and C, which he couldn't do very well at all but had to. Jim likes the new arrangement, enabling him to earn a much higher income. How is this new trading arrangement possible? Because each person now decides to specialize, according to their respective 'comparative advantages.'

Let us now move a step closer to the real world:

(a) Jack is hired by an outside employer to work exclusively on task A, ceding tasks B and C to others.
(b) He does not have to spend time on other lower-productivity tasks—which he was doing earlier before the 'age of specialization.'
(c) With his superior earnings from employment, Jack can now afford to hire outside help to do anything he doesn't want to

do himself. This is the logic of what is called 'Outsourcing'—the rapidly growing modern trend to delegate many erstwhile household chores to third parties.

(d) Nowadays, there is some business outfit ready and willing to carry out any task you care to assign to them, such as childcare, laundering, household cleaning/maintenance, lawn care, cooking, food delivery, personal shopping and so on—the list is almost endless. Such outsourcing enterprises/outfits are springing up everywhere (the task rabbits of the world!).

Without this golden opportunity to 'outsource' those tasks (which you have neither the time nor the inclination to do), our hectic lifestyles would become virtually impossible.

(e) The rapid evolution of modern computer/telephone technology, coupled with the growth of thousands of new web-based businesses, has made possible the adoption of 'outsourcing' as a way of life.

As readers can surmise, the principle of 'comparative advantage' helps everyone to be engaged in activities using their unique skills—multiplying job opportunities and helping to raise incomes and standards of living for all.

The art and science of decision-making is designed to exploit and take advantage of these boundless opportunities; so let us move on and continue our exploration of this exciting decision-landscape.

IV. Making Use of Substitutes
Whenever and wherever an item B can be used in place of another item A to satisfy a certain need, they become substitutes for each other.

A and B need not be perfect substitutes but close enough for most purposes. Indeed, item B may have several substitutes, some of which could be better or more suitable than others.

What does this mean in the context of decision-making?

Whenever item A becomes scarce(more expensive or unavailable), a substitute can take its place. If A suddenly becomes difficult to obtain or commands a much higher price, then B, C or D might serve the same purpose at a lower cost.

For example, many modes of transportation such as plane, boat, train, bus, or taxi can take you from New York to Boston. Suppose commuters usually take the Amtrak train, which costs about $200. If Amtrak hikes the price or cancels its service due to bad weather, you can choose these other alternative modes of transport. Although they may be poor substitutes for Amtrak (you enjoy Amtrak's ambience and convenience), they can still fill the void.

Similarly, whenever your favorite brand of a consumer product (beer, coffee, soda, cereal or whatever) becomes pricey, there is always a close substitute or standby readily available.

When your home entertainment system quits suddenly and unexpectedly, you can entertain yourself in umpteen other ways: listen to radio or recorded music, read a book, play guitar, do crossword puzzles, engage in conversation, visit friends, or just take a walk—whatever you fancy at that moment. Note that such alternative forms of entertainment exist in many forms—limited only by your imagination. The list of potential alternatives is almost endless!

Substitutes exist for anything—almost everywhere, most of the time. It is simply a matter of seeking them out, using your creativity and letting your imagination soar. This is the essence of making choices—finding the 'next best' alternative whenever the preferred item is unavailable. Indeed, throughout history, a great deal of technological progress/innovation took place by finding substitutes (or even creating them outright—as in the case of nylon as substitute for rubber).

V. Supply, Demand and Market Prices

Prices reflect opportunity costs. They also indicate the relative scarcity of an item. At any given time, the forces of supply (quantity available for sale) and demand (someone's willingness and ability to pay) determines the current market price. Buyers compete with one another for scarce resources. When something goes up in price, it signals that supplies are tightening or demand is increasing. Similarly, whenever demand slackens off or supply becomes plentiful, the price goes down.

Smart decision-making involves economizing. This means switching from a more expensive item to a cheaper substitute—serving the same need/purpose. Through this process, everyone ends up conserving resources. Constantly evolving market prices provide the right signals to both producers and consumers, giving incentives to change behavior. The net result is that production and consumption adjust to rapidly changing economic conditions. Short-term price disruptions, though inconvenient, ultimately bring long-term benefits to all.

The emergence of many 'price comparison' websites on the internet has been a boon to consumers in their quest for bargains. The process of buying and selling big-ticket items such as cars, computers, appliances, airline tickets, cruises, vacation packages, hotels and many other products and services has now become less cumbersome. The easier and faster information-gathering process has facilitated decision-making for all.

VI. Implicit and Explicit Costs

It often happens that some of the costs of undertaking an activity are hidden from view or cannot be easily recognized. They may be lurking in the background, distorting your perception of the true (real) cost. Economists call this phenomenon 'implicit costs.' Decisions that don't take 'implicit costs' into account will result in poor allocation of resources and eventually make you 'worse off.'

Many 'Do It Yourself' activities belong to this category. Here are some familiar examples:

(a) You decide to wash your car instead of taking it to the neighborhood car wash facility. You think you can save $15 by doing so. However, the true cost of this 'self-service activity' is the Opportunity Cost of your time + other (material) costs—such as soap, brush, wax, etc. ($10). Let us assume that your wage rate per hour is $25—the value of your time. If washing the car takes one hour, the true total cost becomes $25 + 10 = $35. By personally washing the car you haven't really saved $15: instead, it has cost you $35 ($20 extra!).

Before you protest, let me add that if you enjoy washing the car for fun, diversion, relaxation, exercise, or other reasons, go ahead and do it. But don't be under the illusion that you are saving money by doing so.

Recall the concept of 'comparative advantage.' When Jack and Jim were engaged in doing various chores before starting to trade, both were spending time inefficiently. Their standards of living leapt up many-fold with specialization and trade. The same logic applies to you and me: it makes eminent sense to contract out (outsource) those tasks with hidden (implicit) costs.

Here are other examples of this interesting idea—probably familiar to many readers.

(b) Cut-rate Financing Offer

Vincent had been scouting various banks for a car loan. His Credit Union was recently offering a four-year auto loan at a (low) fixed rate of 1.99%. This special rate was contingent upon using a designated dealer network—a car-buying service. A no-hassle, pre-arranged price was associated with the 1.99% interest rate. Vincent was interested in a Mazda, with a 'sticker price' of about $32,000, which the network was offering at a specific pre-determined price of $30,250—a discount of $1,750 below the list price. Combined with the 1.99% financing, this seemed like a good deal at first.

Before signing on the dotted line, Vincent decided to investigate whether he could find a better deal elsewhere. Indeed, he found an 'internet price' of $28,500—which happened to be $1,750 below the network's 'no hassle' deal.

The relevant question becomes: What is the 'implicit cost' of the Credit Union's offer—the four-year loan @ 1.99% + price tag of $30,250?

As it turned out, Vincent found a 'no strings attached' car loan available at 2.99% elsewhere. Using a financial calculator Vincent figured that the added 1% interest cost would be roughly $1,200. Therefore, buying the car at the internet price of $28,500 would result in saving about $550.

Note: These calculations are entirely based on the specific circumstances cited here. The Credit Union's low interest rate did not compensate for the associated higher-priced car. Caveat: It pays to be skeptical about many such 'cut-rate' offers. One should calculate the true, real, out-of-pocket all-inclusive costs (explicit + implicit) and then make an informed choice.

(c) "An Incredible" Furniture Deal

A well-known furniture store was recently advertising what they termed as a "Very Special Sale." Here is how it read:

"Take 50% off the List Price + pay Delivery Charges (available only for Cash customers)" or "Pay full price with 'free delivery,' interest-free financing is available for up to 4 years for qualified customers. A minimum purchase price of $1,849 is required for this offer."

To evaluate the relative merits of these two options, a prospective customer wondered: 'What is the implicit (hidden) interest cost—of the free-financing offer?'

After making a quick back-of-the-envelope calculation—she figured that the cash option would really cost:

50% of the advertised price: $1,849 = $925

+ Delivery charge $75 = $1,000

The second option (which included free delivery) required regular monthly payments (48 payments, totaling $1,849 over a four-year period). This price difference of $849 (mainly attributable to the interest cost on the four-year loan) implied an interest rate of about 20%.

Decision: She opted for the cash price since she could easily find a far cheaper bank loan at 8.75%!

VII. Sunk Costs

A thorough understanding of the nature of "sunk costs" should help you make sound decisions. Even more important, you will be able to avoid many potential traps. Terms such as "Don't throw good money after bad" or "Let bygones be bygones" aptly sum up the reason why 'sunk costs' should be forgotten and ignored.

The concept refers to any previous action/expenditure that cannot be retrieved or undone and therefore becomes irrelevant. This can happen due to several reasons:

a) A permanent change in the underlying business environment.
b) Rapid technological progress/obsolescence.
c) New government regulations.
d) Changes in climatic conditions, consumer tastes, fashions, etc.

Here is an example to illustrate this phenomenon:

Suppose you bought a state-of-the-art computer two years ago for $5,000 with an expected useful life of five years. A newer model, incorporating much greater speed and many sophisticated features, is now available for $3,000. The older machine has a remaining working life of three years and performs well. You wonder whether you should replace it and buy the newer model.

Is it worth treating the original computer investment as a sunk cost and discard it (or write it off)? Is it economically sensible to buy the new computer?

One way to look at this problem is to consider what you stand to lose by keeping the older computer. It is slower, inefficient, and outdated compared to the new machine (although it still works well). Keeping it is not cost-efficient if 'speed' of computing is a critical consideration. (Its slower speed could result in thousands of hours of wasted time.) Should you discard it in favor of the newer machine, treating it as a sunk cost?

Answer: Although the 'old reliable' can deliver three more years of service, keeping it may not be desirable. If you wait three years to replace it, the opportunity to benefit from all the technological improvements incorporated in the newer machine is lost. This can be problematic. It will cost more money to operate the older machine rather than replacing it. Here is a straightforward calculation to settle the issue.

The Economic Scenario:
Over the next three years, the old computer will cost $1,500 to operate. These costs are attributable to greater power usage, repairs, maintenance, and upkeep ($500 per year x 3). Due to its inferior (slower) performance, it will also require an additional three hundred hours of computing time to do routine tasks relative to the newer model. If your time in front of the computer is worth $40 an hour (the going wage rate for a hired hand), those three hundred hours will cost $12,000 in 'opportunity cost' (or actual wages paid). Thus, the total cost of its operation will amount to $13,500 over the next three years— which is 4.5 times the price of the newer model.

Therefore, selling the 'old reliable' for its salvage value and buying the newer replacement makes eminent economic sense.

Here are some other examples of **sunk costs**. The reluctance to acknowledge them as such is widespread. This causes a great deal of psychological pain and financial loss, which happens all too often.

Last year Jody bought one hundred shares of ABC stock at $50 each. The firm's business has since turned sour, and it is now operating at a loss. There is no prospect of its business recovering and becoming profitable any time soon. The current market price of the stock reflects this reality—$20 per share. If Jody sells her shares, she will register a 'real' loss of $3,000.

Should she get rid of the stock, converting this 'paper loss' into a 'real loss'? Or keep the stock hoping that the business will recover, eventually lifting the stock price? Many stockholders face a similar dilemma!

The answer for Jody is straightforward: sell, take the loss and move on. Her reluctance to admit investment losses (sunk costs) will only compound the problem. Hindsight will not help her, nor do unrealistic hopes and rosy (but false) expectations about the future.

Consider a similar but much less expensive episode.

Sunny feels hungry and decides to order a pizza costing $10. She takes a few bites and discovers that the pizza does not suit her for many reasons: (1) it is too salty, (2) not cooked well, (3) feels rubbery, (4) hard to chew and (5) unappetizing in general. Eating this pizza is going to be problematic. "Should I continue eating or quit?" she wonders. Sunny knows that the price paid is nonrefundable and a replacement is not in the cards.

She decides to head home, leaving the pizza behind. The $10 paid is treated as a sunk cost. It was prudent to discard the food for the sake of her health and future wellbeing.

To drive this point home, I give below some other case studies illustrating the irrelevance of sunk costs.

Let me emphasize that our daily lives are often replete with the common reluctance to admit the reality of sunk costs. This could very well be the result of well-entrenched habits or a lack of appreciation of the harm it inflicts in the long run. Awareness of the concept of sunk costs is central to smart decision-making. This will not only save resources but, more importantly, forestall avoidable future regrets.

The Stahl family had bought 'nonrefundable and non-transferable' airline tickets to their favorite Mexican beach resort. When the day arrived, a family member suddenly fell sick and couldn't get out of bed. They realized that going on the vacation with this health condition would be inadvisable.

In this instance, the money spent on the flights had to be treated as a sunk cost. Though psychologically and financially painful, the Stahls decided to treat it as such.

Note: If the Stahls had purchased either refundable tickets or bought 'trip insurance,' they could have gotten either a full or partial refund, reducing their loss. But this type of hindsight does not help much—after the event!

Priscilla had spent a good deal of time and energy shopping for a fancy dress to wear at the wedding of a close friend. Although she had tried out the outfit earlier, she found it ill-fitting and uncomfortable now. The dress could not be returned, and the price paid was also non-refundable. Rather than ruin her enjoyment of the ball, Priscilla decided to treat the purchase as a 'sunk cost' and donated it to charity. She bought another dress for the wedding party and enjoyed it thoroughly.

The most egregious example of the sunk cost phenomenon is the bleak unemployment picture facing many old-line factory workers—in industries such as coal, steel, textiles, shoes, small electronics, etc. Due to rapid technological changes or shifting world trade patterns, those job skills are rapidly becoming obsolete. Without extensive retraining or relocation, there is no real prospect of these workers regaining their traditional jobs. Moreover, the capital investment (factories, equipment and associated transport facilities) ploughed into these industries may have become permanent casualties of irreversible changes. As such, workers, employers, investors, and policymakers need to address this problem more realistically rather than pour more money and effort to salvage this sinking ship.

VIII. Incentives & Disincentives

Human beings appear to be pre-programmed by nature and also motivated to respond to incentives and disincentives or rewards and punishments. Positive inducements (prizes) and negative ones (sanctions) can often encourage and discourage marked changes in behavior.

They can tip the balance in favor of or against a certain course of action when you are undecided about what to do. Their applications are common and widespread—in fields as varied as agriculture, marketing, finance, healthcare, education, and migration.

This is indeed a fascinating subject, as the following examples will demonstrate.

Myriad examples of everyday decision-making such as when to buy, sell, produce, consume, save, invest, conserve, work, study, exercise, or 'do nothing' at all, are often influenced by incentives/disincentives.

Most people respond, in varying degrees, to the incentive effects of taxes and subsidies. Many research studies have shown that high marginal tax rates can discourage working. Cutting those rates can do the opposite—because of their impact on workers' 'after-tax' earnings.

i) Retirees generally flock to states with low income/sales/property taxes. State governments often give extensive 'tax holidays and tax-exemption status' to employers/firms willing to relocate.

122

ii) Agricultural subsidies are a major policy tool employed by governments throughout the world to encourage local farmers to increase production and discourage imports of certain crops.

iii) Cash incentives such as: refunds, coupons, special holiday discounts, "tax free or duty-free days," etc., induce consumers to buy extra quantities of certain goods and services—spurred by lower prices. Indeed, many families wait for these periodic/seasonal incentives, delaying purchases they already have in mind, until the so-called "bargain days" are announced.

iv) Automobile dealers make frequent use of "promotions/deals" to spur sales—offering (a) special price reductions, (b) cut-rate financing, (c) free maintenance plans, (d) extended warranties, (e) higher trade-in-values, etc., to lure reluctant customers into their showrooms.

Potential buyers who were otherwise not thinking of buying a certain make/model are induced to jump in, eager to take advantage of such special incentives. In a highly competitive market where some automobile manufacturers are struggling to survive, such promotions can clinch a sale.

v) Recently, when sales of a new model just introduced were sagging due to lack of consumer appeal, General Motors offered to buy back the older models at 'higher-than-usual-trade-in- values.' This incentive worked wonders: sales of unsold inventories took off, resulting in a 'shortage' of this newer model!

vi) Purveyors of the tourist industry—airlines, hotels, resorts and cruise lines—use many types of sales incentives/special package deals to fill idle, vacant facilities. Prospective tourists, looking for bargains, are only too happy to take advantage of these promotions—benefiting both sellers and buyers.

vii) Parents of school-going children usually tend to postpone their purchase of school supplies until the annual 'sales tax holiday' takes effect at the end of summer. This window of opportunity is considered a boon when family budgets are especially tight.

viii) Many consumers of alcohol/cigarettes make a point of traveling to neighboring states (which own and operate state-owned liquor stores) to save (or avoid) taxes imposed by their own states. Indeed, vehicles loaded with bulk purchases of these 'tax-free' items can be observed in the crowded parking lots, just across the respective state borders.

6. Government agencies make extensive use of incentive programs:

(a) To encourage farmers to increase production of designated crops, the Federal Agriculture Department offers subsidies based on a certain percentage of output. Those subsidies are withdrawn or cancelled later when supplies have become plentiful and the granaries have been restocked.

(b) Likewise, high tax rates are often imposed periodically to discourage consumption of goods considered harmful to health—such as cigarettes, alcohol, drugs, etc.

(c) Electric utilities make extensive use of 'peak period' pricing to discourage consumption of power during the hottest weeks of the summer season when above-average temperatures can strain their generating capacity. Rebates are also offered to those who voluntarily turn off their air conditioners at predetermined periods. This program works well—it prevents power shut-downs, which would otherwise disrupt normal electricity production.

College Job Placement

Hordes of recruiters (hiring hands) descend on certain college campuses in early Spring—scouting for the best and brightest graduates in specialized fields such as engineering, finance, accounting and information technology—offering special 'sign-up-bonuses.' Indeed, both employers and employees benefit from such incentivized initiatives.

A Philosophical Digression

It is instructive to look at how some ancient Indian philosophers advocated the use of various types of incentives/disincentives to influence human behavior. Their recommendations were designed to elicit an appropriate (favorable) response from recalcitrant individuals.

These techniques are known as Saama, Daana, Bheda and Dhanda—in the (erstwhile) Indian Sanskrit language.

The order in which these incentives (popularly thought of as carrots & sticks) are to be used is critical.

(1) First, one should start with praise/persuasive words to encourage a favorable response.
(2) The second strategy is to shower the individual with plenty of suitable gifts designed to please the recipient and elicit cooperation and compliance. When this strategy fails,
(3) Make use of appropriate intimidation, warnings, threats, and coercion to instill fear of punishment for noncompliance.
(4) (Finally), when all the previous methods have failed, inflict actual punishment to elicit compliance.

Those in authority (such as employers, teachers, parents, or officials) may make judicious use of this four-step program. Its purpose is to secure compliance from recalcitrant individuals. Here is how it works:

First, Engage the Subject with Saama:
This strategy consists of using positive gestures and inducements—such as appropriately chosen words of encouragement and praise, a friendly 'pat on the back' (to boost morale) and appeals to one's cooperative nature. This tactic should work if the subject is sufficiently receptive to praise (ego) and responds favorably. If these sweet-sounding words prove ineffective, you can resort to:

(2) Daana:
You should shower the person with plenty of suitable gifts: money or other desirable objects, promise of future rewards or offer small 'bribes' designed to make the subject do your bidding. If these measures also don't work, then:

(3) Bheda:
Try intimidation, verbal warnings, and threats of punishment.
This strategy is designed to instill fear in the subject's mind. If the person is motivated to avoid physical/psychological pain and suffering, there is a good possibility of compliance. However, if this strategy too fails, then:

(4) Resort to Dhanda, actual punishment—the severity of which may depend on how soon or when the individual decides to comply.

Interestingly, a modern variant of these ancient principles can be found in the operation of the automobile insurance industry. It has the following characteristics, almost in the exact order prescribed, with some variations/modifications:

1. Saama: Rebates and discounts over standard premiums are offered to drivers with good driving records. They may be offered further premium reductions for installing certain speed- monitoring devices.

2. Daana: Rewards or premium discounts are offered for students with good academic grades. Actual reduction of premium is given—contingent on establishing a 'claim-free' history. Drivers who are willing to undergo certain 'driver education/safe driving courses' may become eligible for extra discounts.

3. Bheda: Threats of premium increases are routine for those who do not maintain a satisfactory driving record. Warnings are issued for those with repeated traffic violations, speeding citations or minor accidents/claims. Notices of potential non-renewal or policy cancellations are also common.

4. Dhanda: Prohibitive premium increases and eventual cancellation of coverage for repeated violations/accidents. (Without insurance coverage, it is illegal to operate an automobile. This can become a real hardship for most drivers.)

Decision Time:

For another application of these principles—praise, gifts, warnings and punishment (in a typical American household)—one may observe how some parents try to influence their children's behavior. Which one of these strategies is appropriate will depend on the personality of your youngster.

Here is the typical scenario:
Johnny has still not completed his unfinished homework due tomorrow morning. He has been sulking, dillydallying, and spending time watching his favorite TV show. At this point, his mother tries several tactics to motivate him:

First: she invokes Saama: "Honey, it is really an easy exercise to finish. I know you can do it in a jiffy. Start right now and you will be happy when it's done. Afterwards, you can watch the TV show until bedtime."

Second: Daana: "If (and when) you finish the homework I will give you a special treat—you are really going to like it." (The anticipation of the special gift is designed to elicit a positive response.)

Third: Frustrated with Johnny's inaction, Mother threatens him with Bheda: "If you don't do your homework right away, I am going to cut off this week's allowance. You will be grounded; you cannot invite your friend Sam over this weekend."

Still, Johnny sulks; he remains unconvinced by Mother's threat.

Finally, she resorts to Dhanda: "Go and sit in the corner until I give you permission to move. No TV or your favorite chocolate dessert today."

To summarize:
One of the most effective and least expensive motivators is verbal praise and/or admonition, depending on the context. Words can have a powerful impact on people's behavior/reactions: either to strive harder or slacken their efforts. A friendly pat on the back, a word of encouragement, a simple gesture of true appreciation can often elicit the desired

response to carry out a task expeditiously. Those in positions of power or authority (such as employers, administrators, teachers, leaders, or parents) certainly understand the efficacy of positive and negative incentives. Everyone likes to be appreciated when they are doing a good job, thereby boosting their sense of self-esteem. Regardless of age, gender or other personal characteristics, people enjoy hearing words of praise for a job well done. Likewise, one way to discourage people from doing their best is to keep pointing out their mistakes and failures—creating resentment and ill-will.

Importance of Role Models

It is often said that a 'picture is worth a thousand words.'

Similarly, setting a good example (being a 'role model') works wonders to inspire others—an indirect and powerful way to influence decision-making.

Youngsters of impressionable age like to imitate those whom they truly admire. Anyone in a position of leadership (influencers?) can put this invisible power to great advantage. Stories of dedicated/great teachers who have inspired their students to reach high levels of achievement and excellence are legendary. You may fondly recall how a certain charismatic leader, speaker, teacher, friend, boss or mentor gently prodded you to try and succeed at something that you thought you could never do. There is magic in this hidden power of words to persuade those who are afraid to venture into the unknown. If you are inspired to try and put forth the requisite effort, the decision may well turn to be very rewarding.

IX. The Law of Diminishing Returns

There are certain economic principles that stand out and have universal appeal and validity. One of these is the Law of Diminishing Returns. Simply stated, this theory asserts that additional or repeated applications of a variable input (such as hours of labor), in conjunction with another fixed input (such as an acre of land), will eventually result in slower growth of output. Stated differently, one cannot expect a linear relationship between inputs and output without a change in the underlying technology of production.

This theory is of enormous importance in making decisions. It tells you how much energy should be expended in doing something: you reach a point beyond which extra units of effort will become uneconomical. In the language of economics, the marginal (extra) benefit will fall short of marginal cost. When you reach that point, one should redirect resources to other uses rather than persist.

Here are some examples or applications:

i) As you continue to squeeze (apply physical power) to a honeycomb or citrus fruit, you will get progressively smaller quantities of honey (or juice). No matter how hard you squeeze, the yield continues to dwindle.

ii) A 'perfect diamond' will cost twice or thrice as much as a 'slightly imperfect' one. This is because cutting, polishing and shaping the diamond to make it 'perfect' (or appear flawless) costs enormous amounts of time and effort.

iii) Here is a useful tip for diamond shoppers: A 0.97- or 0.98-ct. diamond can be a 'best buy' in terms of price and quality vis-à-vis a

1-ct. diamond. The infinitesimal difference in quality will be hardly noticeable while the big price difference can hit your pocketbook very hard!

iv) Picking 'low-hanging fruits' is easily accomplished compared to climbing up the tree to reach those hard-to-reach branches.

v) Many species of insects, birds and animals instinctively seem to know how to apply the least amount of effort to get the maximum feeding output.

vi) Bees and butterflies feed on easily accessible supplies of nectar in a flower and then quickly move on to the next plentiful source rather than wasting time trying to get the last drop out of each previously visited source. Grazing animals too keep moving from one field to the next in search of 'greener pastures' in adjacent fields. Most predators seem to know when and how to pounce on their prey for the quickest kill—and equally important—when to give up the chase without undue expenditure of precious time and energy. (This is a process of learning by doing—through repeated trials and errors—but they seem to learn fast.)

vii) The pursuit of perfection—in many fields of endeavor—is not for the faint of heart. The requisite effort can become overly burdensome. Counter-intuitive as this may seem, ignoring the Law of Diminishing Returns can cost you dearly in the end: the marginal benefits seldom justify the associated marginal costs.

X. The Marginal Principle

Regardless of the actual level or quantity of any asset you possess, it is those small or incremental changes taking place (either up or down) that influence decisions. This is also true of your psychic wellbeing on a day-to-day basis.

Consider the state of your health. If you enjoy good health, the onset of a cold, small accident or injury will upset you and make you feel unhappy and miserable. On the other hand, if you were suffering from prolonged illness, a sudden small improvement can make you feel much happier and put you in a good mood.

If you are a high-achieving student always getting good grades, just one 'C' this semester can upset you. For an average 'C' student, getting a single 'B' can bring great joy.

If your stock portfolio has been doing well and you suddenly happen to have a loss, your mood can become gloomy. However, a series of 'down days' followed by a single upward swing can bring enormous relief.

Your relationships too follow this principle. A generally harmonious relationship with a loved one can become tainted with a small misunderstanding or quarrel. However, if you don't particularly enjoy your present relationship, a sudden unexpected act of kindness or demonstration of love can change your mood for the better. A kind word, a small gesture of appreciation can work wonders to bring sunshine into a souring marriage.

Unless you are 'super rich,' getting a small bonus or cash award/prize can make you feel richer. For a wage-earner just getting by, losing or misplacing a few bucks can be painful. An indigent person will feel momentarily rich when they find a dollar bill on the road.

If you are always well fed, just one day of experiencing the pangs of hunger can become somewhat unpleasant. A constantly hungry person feels overjoyed if she can get few morsels of bread.

Anyone experiencing constant pain will feel a great deal of relief as soon as an aspirin/Tylenol helps to provide temporary pain relief. On the other hand, a few abrasions on your skin caused by some minor injury can put you in a bad mood.

Here is the broad take-away from these examples:

It is not the actual 'level' of any entity you possess that determines your prevailing mood or behavior but slight changes or fluctuations thereof, either up or down. You are constantly reminded of the 'marginal changes' taking place in the environment you inhabit.

XI. Production Externalities

There are innumerable occasions in everyday life when one person's choices and actions can result in some unexpected, unintended, and unavoidable (external) impact on others. The resulting outcomes may be either beneficial (desirable) or harmful (undesirable).

Such interactions emanate (i) either from the physical proximity of the parties involved or (ii) some other technological/environmental inter-relationships that are embedded in those activities. Such 'side-effects,' whenever and wherever they occur, are known as "externalities"— beyond the control of the decision-maker.

Such externalities can be a blessing or a curse, depending on circumstances. To understand and appreciate their pervasiveness, I give below some interesting examples:

(a) Mary enjoys gardening. She spends a great deal of time and effort growing beautiful flowers and fragrant herbs/plants in her yard. Their beauty and fragrance can be enjoyed by all her neighbors. They derive many unexpected external benefits from

Mary's gardening. Those beautiful flowers provide a feast for the eyes of all passersby. The gentle breezes wafting elegant fragrances emanating from Mary's garden fill the entire neighborhood air. In short, her garden confers immense 'external benefits' on her neighbors without any special effort on her part. She feels proud and happy about it.

Notice that this beneficial effect is associated with the nature (production technology) of gardening. Mary's neighbors can reap a bonanza without her explicit permission or knowledge. Nor can she prevent this externality from taking place.

(b) A famous example of this phenomenon was first brought to our attention by the Nobel Economist Ronald Coase. His seminal contribution was to explain how one entity, quietly going about its own business, can indirectly (unintentionally) help or hurt another—without intending to do so!

Here is the scenario Coase described:
Two neighbors, a beekeeper and a florist, live and work side by side. The bees, in their quest for nectar from the abundant flowers, also pollinate them. This interactive process confers an external benefit on the florist, who can now grow and harvest a bumper crop of flowers without any additional effort. The garden's proximity to the beehives makes this externality possible.

Similarly, the abundance of nectar in the flower garden provides ample food for the bees, thus increasing honey production for the beekeeper. This 'good or beneficial' externality springs from a technological (production) relationship—in this case, because both flower growing and honey production occur side by side.

(c) Professor Coase also provided a remarkable example of a 'bad, harmful or undesirable' externality. A pristine idyllic village is located near a busy railroad. The village existed there long before the railroad came along. Many trains pass through that neighborhood frequently, whistling, bellowing, and emitting smoke into the clean air. The resulting noise and air pollution is harming the villagers. Their relatively tranquil life is disturbed by the operation of the railroad. Neither the village nor the railroad can coexist without this undesirable side-effect—an unintended externality brought about by the technology of railroad operation.

Unlike the previous example, in this case the harm is one-sided; the 'external cost' of noise and air pollution is shifted on the village residents with no corresponding benefit to the railroad.

Note that the railroad did not intend to cause any harm to the villagers. Yet that is precisely what happens when the trains pass by. This is a classic example of what is known as 'market failure'—situations where people pursuing their preferred activities are unable to prevent spillover effects on third parties.

Such situations provide the rationale for government intervention—regulations to modify/mitigate as much as possible—those harmful, unwanted spillover effects resulting from private economic activity and ordinary market transactions.

To achieve this result, the economic landscape should have in place a well-designed system of controls such as public ordinances, rules, regulations, licensing, permits, appropriate incentives and disincentives. The system should be designed to encourage activities that generate beneficial externalities while also trying to minimize those with undesirable spillovers.

Decision-makers in the public arena have a great responsibility to legislate and implement policies that promote these twin objectives.

XI. Consumption Externalities

People engaged in their everyday activities make decisions that they hope will promote their own personal interests. One doesn't normally know nor think about how those decisions impact third parties in unexpected ways. As we have seen, when people live and work near each other, what one person chooses to do can have spill-over effects on their neighbors. Those effects may be short-lived or can sometimes last over much longer periods. Similarly, the side-effects could be merely local or spread over larger areas. (Ocean pollution and smoke from Canadian wildfires spreading over wide areas of USA are illustrative of this phenomenon.)

Here are some typical examples of consumer externalities.

(i) Shopping trips on holidays or busy weekends often result in shortage of parking space for everybody. Some drivers choose to go round and round, looking for empty parking spaces, which may be nonexistent or hard to find. They spend much time doing so and create hazards for other motorists.

(ii) Driving automobiles on congested highways during peak hours imposes long delays on fellow motorists and creates environmental pollution.

(iii) When people crowd up on the beaches during the hot summer months, you are left with less space for yourself and your family.

(iv) Some drivers habitually turn on their radios and loudspeakers at high volume, blasting their favorite music, while threatening the tranquility of others.

(v) When tourists visiting the National Parks forget to clean up their act, they cause much inconvenience and discomfort to fellow visitors.

(vi) Cell phone users talking loudly in public places, shopping centers, theaters, and restaurants unwittingly cause noise pollution—irritating and disturbing the peace of those sitting nearby.

(vii) (You may have noticed that it has become standard practice for many such establishments to announce that patrons should turn off their electronic devices.)

And the list goes on. What can be done to mitigate these undesirable consumer externalities?

There are solutions—both simple and complex.

As we have seen, there is a strong case for public policy intervention to minimize or prevent some harmful externalities. Familiar examples are air and water pollution causing environmental degradation and the health hazards of certain economic activities.

The unmistakable implication is the paramount need for everyone to take these externalities into account whenever and wherever possible, and act responsibly.

Exercising care and restraint and forcing oneself to be constantly aware of the repercussions of your decisions on third parties is the first important step.

Next, activities that produce beneficial externalities should be promoted and encouraged. Activities causing harmful externalities should be discouraged, curtailed or, in rare cases, even prohibited (such as smoking in public areas).

Third, widespread use of protocols that automatically help us to promote the 'common good' should be established and/or encouraged.

Here is a partial list, already familiar to most readers.

a) Establish 'no-smoking' zones.
b) Enforce the 'first-come-first-served' rule.
c) 'Yield' signs at busy road intersections.
d) Restricted/limited parking time on busy streets.
e) 'Handicapped Only' signs in parking lots.
f) People using wheelchairs get priority access everywhere.
g) Fines/penalties for violation of rules in National Parks.
h) 'Dogs on leash' and 'Clean up after your pets' signs with warnings.
i) Mandatory inoculations against communicable diseases.

Since decisions by individuals/businesses do not automatically take account of the presence of externalities, it becomes incumbent on governmental/public bodies to intervene, with the object of modifying certain 'market-determined' outcomes. This is the rationale and justification for introducing certain types of taxes (to discourage) and subsidies (to encourage) targeted activities. Likewise, appropriate rules and regulations, restrictions and even outright prohibitions are called for in areas involving public health and the environment—to promote the wellbeing of all citizens.

Rather than belaboring this point, let me add some useful guidelines for all decision-makers.

1. Think about the potential impact of your actions on others—neighbors, coworkers, employers, employees, future generations, the environment, etc., and act accordingly in everybody's best interests.

2. 'Do No Harm' to others should be the watchword guiding all your decisions.

3. Whenever possible, try to educate yourselves about the existence and potential impact of different types of externalities.
4. Try practicing the Golden Rule—"Do unto others as you would have them do unto you."

A Summing Up

It is now time to weave together these diverse concepts—akin to putting together the different strands of pearls in a necklace. To facilitate this task, I offer a comprehensive example based on trends in modern suburban living.

The spread of housing communities located in concentric circles around big central cities such as New York, Boston, Los Angeles, Chicago, Houston, and Washington, D.C., demonstrates the application of many interesting economic principles.

In recent years, the availability of 'park-n-ride' facilities, strategically located near commuter railroad stations (called metro parks), has made it possible for thousands of city workers to buy homes in distant suburbs (or exurbs) at so-called 'affordable prices.' Housing is generally cheaper, the farther away it is located from the downtown hubs. However, the long commuting distance can be a real hardship. For suburbanites, driving on the congested beltways and byways to reach the central city during peak working hours can be a great challenge. Older parking facilities surrounding many downtown office buildings simply don't have enough space to accommodate all the potential commuters. Besides, the associated road congestion, traffic delays and environmental pollution create a host of undesirable externalities.

Imaginative urban planning has partly solved many of these problems. People who live in the new suburban neighborhoods can drive to their closest 'park-n-ride' facility and park their vehicle at a nominal cost (often subsidized by the local municipal governments) in a safe and secure place. These large multi-storied parking structures are constructed adjacent to the metro train stations. The commuters then board the trains and have a leisurely trip headed to the city.

These arrangements have helped to reduce a host of undesirable externalities—road congestion, high gasoline consumption and car pollution.

Figure 8: Growth of Suburbs around Central City

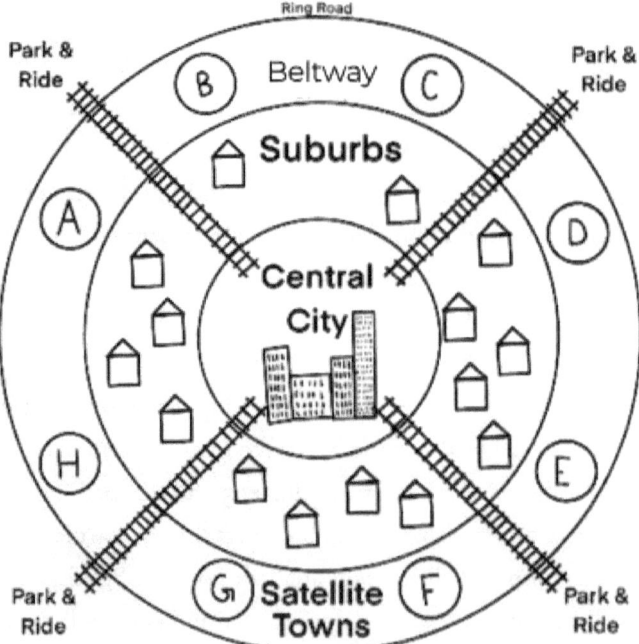

Here, in a nutshell, one can see the multiple benefits of these arrangements:

i. The suburban commuters can afford better housing (amenities such as more living space, lower housing costs/rents and a more pleasing (leafy) residential environment).

ii. Those who still prefer to live in central city neighborhoods, to be closer to their places of work, are also presumably better off. Because of the dispersion of the population to the suburbs, city residents can now enjoy the perceived comforts/conveniences of city dwelling. Presumably their rents have gone down too, thanks to the suburban exodus.

   (It is conceivable that housing costs/rents as well as overcrowding/congestion in central cities would have been far greater without this population dispersion.)

iii. The suburbanites have apparently decided to substitute extra housing space and a more desirable living environment in place of proximity to work. This 'trade-off' comes at a significant cost in terms of commuting time.

iv. Thus, the construction of 'park-n-ride' facilities, coupled with the availability of mass public transit systems (wherever they exist), has significantly impacted people's residential choices. It has undoubtedly helped to reduce congestion and the cost of living in central cities as well as the suburbs. Everybody is presumably better off as a result, improving their overall quality of life.

v. As readers can appreciate, this case study demonstrates how certain core economic concepts such as scarcity, supply-and-demand, trade-offs, opportunity costs, substitutes, incentives, and externalities form an integral part of making everyday decisions.

XIII. Cost-Benefit Analysis

We now introduce the concept of 'cost-benefit analysis,' a tool used to evaluate whether a proposed course of action is desirable/worthwhile.

Before carrying out major decisions (sometimes even minor ones), it is important to look at all their potential costs and consequences—in as much detail as possible. The effort spent in doing so will pay rich dividends. The process will ensure adoption of worthy projects (decisions) while eschewing potentially harmful ones.

What types of costs and benefits are we talking about? It depends on the nature of the problem. Sometimes they are easy to identify, quantify and evaluate. At other times this effort can be very time-consuming, challenging, frustrating and difficult—most probably all of the above!

Some of the costs and benefits will not be obvious at first. This should not discourage you from carefully seeking them out. On the contrary, stepping up your efforts to get hold of them is essential. Eventually this effort can save you a lot of psychic pain and regrets. Knowing in advance whether the decision makes sense, renders it easier to implement and ensure its eventual success.

Costs and benefits may be explicit as well as implicit. The latter (hiding in the background and difficult to identify/assess) should be sought out and accounted for. Otherwise, a distorted picture will emerge, rendering the whole exercise questionable.

The various costs and benefits must be classified in terms of their potential impact on your future wellbeing and quality of life. For example, ask yourself:

How is this decision going to affect/change my life?

i. Is it going to improve my financial situation? How? When? By how much? What if the expected results do not materialize?

ii. What will be its impact on my physical/emotional/psychic health? Will this decision make me feel more relaxed, relieved, happier, more content and able to enjoy life better? Can I get greater control over the 'problems' that are vexing me now? How will the decision 'solve' these issues and bring psychological/mental relief?

iii. Can it bring about a change in my social standing? If so, how?

iv. Will this decision impact my spiritual life in any way? For better or worse?

While some decisions are followed by quick results, others will take time to come to fruition. These delayed flows of benefits and costs may be sorted out into three categories:

(a) short-term—days, weeks, months, a year or two.

(b) medium-term—2 to 5 years.

(c) long-term—5+ years.

In some cases, decisions made today will have far-reaching consequences for many years, probably stretching over your entire lifetime (think of education, career choices, marriage, investments, relocation, migration, etc.).

I. Short-term

The effects of routine, day-to-day decisions wear off quickly. Such decisions are usually repetitive, such as:

Grocery purchases/consumer goods and services.

Medical/dental consultations/treatments.

Shopping for entertainment, socializing.

Participation in sports and recreational activities.

As you can see, most such decisions are habitual, automatic, and repetitive. Therefore, one need not spend a great deal of time and effort in thinking about them.

II. Medium-term

Examples of 'medium-term' decisions are:

Purchase of household appliances, home repairs, replacements.

Buying and selling of automobiles/vehicles.

Travel and vacations.

Income-oriented investments and financial transactions.

These types of decisions generally have a longer 'time horizon' and may also involve significant financial outlays; their impact on the family budget can be significant.

III. Long-term

The effects of longer-term decisions, such as college education, job/career choices, marriage/divorce, child rearing, house buying/ selling, certain critical healthcare choices and retirement-based investments, can stretch over decades—indeed, one's lifetime. They require deep reflection and careful analysis. Rushing into such decisions without a thorough cost-benefit analysis is inadvisable.

Finally, there is a class of decisions known as irrevocable or irreversible which, once made, cannot be altered. Examples of these are:

(a) setting up and operating certain financial/charitable trusts.
(b) critical medical/health-related choices.
(c) organ transplants/donations.
(d) retirement decisions, including disbursement of pensions/annuities and Social Security.

Estimation Bias:
There are three types of biases that can distort your cost-benefit analysis. These are:

(a) Underestimation of costs
(b) Overestimation of benefits
(c) Improper accounting

At times it so happens that there is a natural tendency to gloss over some inconvenient future costs as well as to exaggerate some perceived benefits.

This frequently happens because of some hidden, unspecified eagerness to act or an unconscious tendency to justify certain decisions to yourself (or others). Such biases are common whenever you are anxious to reap some quick psychological rewards and gloss over unexplored costs that can emerge much later.

A personal note: I have observed some folks casually indulging in such behavioral patterns—much to their future regret. They were overeager to go ahead with what they wanted to do regardless of future costs/consequences. Here are some common, everyday examples:

i. Engage in relentless gossip: Rationale: "It is pretty harmless and certainly entertaining, don't you agree? Everyone does it."

ii. Have a few more drinks: "I can definitely handle it; I have been working all day with some very difficult people and need to relax a bit."

iii. Help yourself with generous quantities of pastries or desserts, despite the doctor's warning: "This is an occasion to celebrate; it comes rarely and besides, these goodies are irresistible!"

iv. Drive under the influence: "There are very few vehicles on the road; no one is in plain sight, and I am really sober."

v. Justify purchasing an expensive, hot-selling new gadget: "The older model is too slow and is acting up. I will have bragging rights before anyone else."

vi. One of the most common examples of underestimation concerns distances and/or driving time: "I will be there in half an hour," although it can easily take twice as much time under normal circumstances.

Does this type of behavior seem familiar? You may not even think of these as 'decisions' since they are often unconscious, habitual, automatic, or instantaneous reactions to some external stimuli.

Another variation on this theme: When the potential benefits of an action take a long time to come to fruition, the underlying effort may seem daunting, too time-consuming, or not worth doing.

For example, when a doctor-recommended regimen of diet and exercise take many months to show promising (visible) results, some people tend to give up too early. On the other hand, sponsors of advertisements such as 'Lose 20 lbs. in 30 days or your money back' have no trouble finding plenty of eager takers willing to pay up front. Presumably, people find the long-term regimen's 'psychic' costs (slow-acting remedies) much more painful than those upfront financial outlays.

Youngsters who sulk when asked to do household chores or tend to put off doing homework assignments until the last minute (behavior-patterns familiar to many parents) are classic examples of this tendency.

Cost-benefit analysis, when earnestly and diligently carried out, can be productive of good results and also financially rewarding.

Chapter V

Case Studies of Smart Decision-making

Having collected the various nuts and bolts of the decision-making framework, it is instructive to bring them together. Recall the discussion of 'triggering mechanisms' discussed earlier.

To illustrate, here are some typical situations:

(a) Leslie thinks it is time to settle a divorce suit she had filed many years ago, which remains unresolved. She believes an out-of-court-settlement is feasible/desirable and will help to reduce the lingering uncertainty. She asks her lawyer to move ahead with this new plan.

(b) Alex has concluded, after months of appeals, that it is preferable to pay a fine/penalty instead of continuing to contest an IRS tax-deficiency notice.

(c) Tom has been feeling uncomfortable about a long-standing dispute with his neighbor. He wants to restore cordial neighborly relations and is offering a generous compromise plan, which he hopes will settle the issue.

Note: While these individuals have found ways to resolve festering issues, there are others where the subjects are unsure about what to do. They typify underlying conflicts, which need to be resolved (see Chapter VI).

(d) Jacob is planning to retire in three years, when he reaches the mandatory retirement age. His employer is currently offering a 'severance package' to some employees, to induce early retirement. He wonders whether to accept the offer or opt out. "Wouldn't I be better off if I work a while longer and thereby become eligible for a bigger pension? Wouldn't that ensure a more comfortable lifestyle?" He feels conflicted because his wife thinks he should take the offer now and quit.

(e) Richard is facing a real conflict about which celebratory party he should attend: He is unable to make up his mind, because he thinks every one of them is equally deserving of his presence: (i) the wedding anniversary of his cousin, (ii) the graduation of his brother's daughter, (iii) the retirement party for a long-term colleague.

(f) Which mayoral candidate should I vote for? Each one of them seem equally worthy of support.

The essence of this type of problem or dilemma is a conflict, which needs to be addressed. A definite choice must be made among competing alternatives. Doing one thing rules out another, an equally desirable choice. Which one will result in the least amount of subsequent 'regret'?

What steps should be followed to assess these alternatives and then make an informed selection?

What are the respective costs and benefits of each available option? What types of consequences, desirable and undesirable, will emanate from each choice?

These individuals must ponder their puzzling questions carefully, make their choices and then be prepared to accept whatever consequences ensue.

This is the essence of 'making up your mind'—and learning how to resolve various underlying conflicts.

Having explained the nature of these decision situations, let us now proceed to look at their salient features:

1. There is a strong triggering mechanism.
2. The goal of the decision is clearly articulated.
3. The decision reflects a commitment to move away from the status quo. There is a clear recognition of the need for resources to carry out the stated mission. The proposed action plan demonstrates a willingness/readiness to find and deploy those resources.
4. The action plan is followed by a timeline to get the mission accomplished.
5. There is a recognition of the opportunity costs and trade-offs involved in carrying out the decision.
6. A detailed cost-benefit analysis of the proposed action has been completed. The expected benefits will justify incurring the costs associated with the preferred course of action.
7. The decision-maker is aware of, willing and able to shoulder some risks in carrying out the decision. Otherwise, no progress/resolution is possible.

The Paramount Need for Setting Clearly Stated Goals:

The first, most basic step in making effective decisions is to think clearly about the goal you want to accomplish. The goal should be defined in specific, concrete, measurable terms.

Vague wishes or hopes for a better, more meaningful life, such as "I want to be rich, famous, healthy, happy, successful" do not suffice. These are not very helpful guides to action. Though worthy and desirable, they are neither specific nor measurable. Such statements are like lines drawn in the sand: they keep shifting randomly and aimlessly. Soon they become blurred and invisible. Therefore, one must have well-defined, specific goals so that you can look back and see whether you were successful in accomplishing them.

By way of illustration, I present below some case studies of subjects who have clearly articulated goals. They are drawn from different walks of life, pinpoint what they have in mind and demonstrate how they came up with the appropriate decision.

(a) Improving Physical Health

Roy, a middle-aged family man, is overweight by almost fifty pounds. He is not comfortable with his current weight and appearance. He is unable to walk for fifteen minutes without feeling tired and exhausted. He knows he is terribly out of shape and is determined to change his ways. He wants to become physically fit, trimmer and to bring down his high blood pressure. He sets the following goal for himself:

"I am not satisfied with my current BMI (body mass index—a measure of fatty tissues, usually measured around the waist). I have gotten myself into this unhealthy condition due to my bad eating habits and lack of exercise. I need to change my present unhealthy lifestyle. My doctor has strongly urged me to do so. Starting now I am going to lose four pounds every month and will continue doing so for the next twelve months. I think this is realistic and achievable. I will start a regimen of daily workout for 45 minutes and stick to the diet program recommended by my nutritionist. I will monitor my progress every week. I am taking a photograph of myself today and will keep doing so every month until I reach my goal."

(b) Diabetes Management
Here is the goal Amanda set for herself on Mother's Day:

"I have been lax in keeping my blood sugar level under control. My daughter has been nagging me about this problem since last May. I remember telling her then that I will take care of myself but haven't done so. Today being Mother's Day, I want my children to know that their mother is determined to monitor her blood sugar regularly every day. I will bring down my present A1C level (a measure of glucose in the bloodstream) down from 8.7 to 7.5 –a realistic goal—within the next three months. After reaching that goal, I must continue to keep it at that lower level, permanently. My doctor had warned me about the dangers of high A1C levels during my last physical checkup and had made concrete recommendations to bring it down.

"Unfortunately, I did not follow through. To reach my goal, I will gradually cut down on sweets, candy, desserts, and soda. I realize this is going to be difficult and rather painful psychologically because I have a sweet tooth. Still, I am now convinced that there is no other easier alternative. This plan will be put into place starting today. I know my children will be happy to know about my resolve."

(c) A Variation on This Theme: Yoga Classes
Laura, an avid reader, was impressed by the description of the benefits of yoga when she read Elizabeth Gilbert's book **Eat, Pray, Love**. Gilbert writes that her experiences in a yoga retreat in India transformed her

outlook on life, in more ways than one. She touts the benefits of yoga as a very effective way to get control over one's body, mind, and spirit.

Says Laura: "My physical therapist has been telling me for months that after I finish my current therapy sessions, I should enroll in a yoga class to gain abdominal strength and greater flexibility with my limb movements. Recently, I also read some articles extolling the many benefits of 'alternative therapies' such as yoga and acupuncture. So as soon as my physical therapy sessions are over, I will start doing yoga. If needed, I can also supplement this with acupuncture (on a trial basis). I have filled out an enrollment form for the yoga sessions at the local Y, beginning next September."

Financial Goals

(a) Funds for a Mediterranean Cruise
The Jenkins want to take a Mediterranean cruise to commemorate their 10th Wedding Anniversary. They have a concrete plan to accomplish this goal.

"We must save at least $5,000 by Christmas next year to have sufficient funds to pay for the ten-day cruise. Based on the Cruise Line's brochure, we need to come up with four grand for a cabin with a balcony and full sea view. To pay for this, we are setting up a vacation fund to which we will automatically transfer $250 every month. This should grow into $5,000 in twenty months' time. We figured that taking the cruise is more important than other types of spending—such as movies, casinos, restaurants, and maid service. We can live without those little luxuries for a while—our new priority calls for some readjustment of the monthly budget."

(b) Reducing Debt Burden

Katy, a single mother with mounting credit card balances, has decided on the following plan of action to get rid of her debt within the next two years.

"This credit card balance of $4,850 is hanging heavily on my head. I was not careful in managing my finances. Recent notices from the debt collector have been a wakeup call, really. I must address this problem immediately. I can't get a good night's sleep worrying about this debt. I want to wipe it out completely. I was planning to buy a new car because my ten-year-old jalopy breaks down frequently and has become unreliable. As long as I have this credit card debt, I cannot get a decent car loan. My present FICO score is only about 650, making me ineligible for a low-interest loan, which many banks are currently offering. I don't want to take, nor can I afford, another loan right now. I am tired of paying high interest rates. Before I apply for a car loan, I must pay off all my credit card debt. To do so, I plan to increase my monthly installment debt payments.

"The bank rate calculator I consulted tells me that to reach my goal, I must start paying $230 per month. This means an extra $75 over and above my current installments. This will be a stretch—but I must find the extra money by eliminating some other discretionary spending. I will stop buying new clothes until this debt is cleared up."

(c) Accumulating Retirement Funds

Amanda, a high school teacher, consulted a financial adviser to see where she stood with respect to her retirement planning. She wants to make sure that the money she has put into the teachers' retirement fund would carry her through her golden years when she retires at age 67.

She is not sure of this yet; she has heard several retired teachers make remarks such as:

"I wish I had contributed more money to my 401(k) plan during my working years. I made a big mistake by not forcing myself to do so. Now I find myself terribly under-funded; I am afraid I will run out of money in the next few years. Afterwards, I could face a bleak financial future."

Such remarks from retired colleagues frightened Amanda. She decided to raise her contributions to 10% of her gross salary, instead of the current 8% rate. Her adviser applauded her decision; she now feels comfortable with the revised plan.

(d) Mortgage Refinancing

The Rouse family has been toying with the idea of refinancing their current thirty-year fixed-rate mortgage. They want to take advantage of the prevailing low interest rate environment. They had been putting off this decision mainly due to inertia. They kept saying: "We will do it soon. There is still plenty of time."

Recently they heard some expert's comment on the TV that mortgage rates were likely to go up after the election. They panicked—but decided to make a move right away. They drew up a viable refinancing plan. Their reasoning was:

"Our current mortgage rate of 8% is higher than what is available in the market right now. With an excellent FICO score of 785, we should be able to get a better rate—in the range of 5.7%-5.8%. This should save us at least $150 per month even after paying 'closing costs' of about $3,200 for the refinance. Here is a great window of opportunity to redirect the resulting savings to increase contributions to our IRAs and build up funds for retirement. We can thus 'kill two birds with one stone.'"

Accordingly, the Rouses have marked their calendar for an appointment with the mortgage bank.

Professional Goals

(e) The Ambitious/Aspiring Author

Rachel is working on a manuscript for her book, tentatively titled: 'The Hunting Strategy of Predatory Birds'. She has signed a contract with a publisher that is fast approaching the deadline set earlier. She is not satisfied with her progress with the manuscript.

Rachel is determined to complete the writing as soon as practicable. Her other duties and responsibilities as a teacher are delaying the project. She has come up with a revised submission plan for the book.

She says: "I should be able to complete the first draft within the next four months, before the summer season rolls in. Then I can enjoy the family vacation we have planned—without worrying about the unfinished book project.

"Toward that end, I plan on completing the remaining part of the field research within the next two months. This should be followed by preparing a first draft, which I estimate will take about two months. I am going to write a minimum of four to six pages every day; this target is practical and achievable, given my current work schedule.

"The next task of reviewing and reworking the draft, I estimate, will take another two months. So, I think I can finish the manuscript before packing for the summer vacation, which I am eagerly looking forward to."

If, due to some unforeseen circumstances, Rachel cannot stick to this schedule, she plans to take a leave of absence from teaching for a few weeks. Completing the book project and getting it published is her highest priority right now!

Business Goals

(a) Let us take a close look at the new production plan that Frank, the manufacturer of a small power tools outfit, has come up with, to revive sagging sales:

"We should aim for a minimum of fifty sales calls every day to generate customer interest in our newly remodeled drills. Sales agents will be asked to step up their contacts by at least 10% above current levels so that the targeted market penetration can be achieved. If this effort bears fruit, we should be able to increase our annual revenues by about $5 million (before the next fiscal year rolls around). We will commit an additional $25,000 over and above our current marketing budget, if necessary, to reach this goal. We can also provide additional budgetary resources to reward those sales agents who achieve or exceed their assigned quotas. They will welcome this extra incentive!

"Our newly designed and superior drills, priced competitively, should interest our loyal customers, as well as induce new ones to our showrooms.

"Our commitment to quality, dedicated service, and product warranties should help us to meet our sales projections."

(b) Jeremy, a recent college graduate and an aspirant for the legal profession, has set himself the following goal:

"My plan is to pass the Bar examination before age 25. To accomplish this, I will review the last five years of syllabi/examinations and study the topics contained therein. I must devote about three hours daily to do the library research needed to do this. It would also be helpful to consult the 'Litigation Review' and 'Corporate Law Research Manuals' since I am going to specialize in this area.

"Starting now, my daily work schedule should accommodate this plan. Although this requires a great deal of adjustments/cutbacks in my other commitments, I am ready for it. I want to be at the top of my field in five years, enabling me to earn $200,000 annually. I realize that newly minted lawyers have a hard time making a decent living, but I am determined to beat those odds.

(c) Cosmetic Distribution Agent:
Consider what Mary, a sales agent for a large perfume manufacturer, has to say about her plans to sharply reduce her bloated inventory (ordered earlier in anticipation of holiday sales, which did not pan out).

"My plan is to reduce the accumulated inventory of unsold items within the next three months. To do so, I will recruit two additional sales agents. Last year, our 'net interest payments on receivables owed'—a measure of money tied up in inventories—was almost $50,000. I cannot afford this huge carrying cost. It is reducing my profit margins below industry standards—a minimum of 25% on invested capital.

"Following the action plan discussed with my suppliers, I will advertise and offer a 'one-time 20% promotional discount' to all new customers over and above our current loyalty program. Hopefully, this new incentive should move our unsold inventories quickly.

"Further, to attract potential younger customers, we will offer a surprise gift package if they agree to buy a minimum of $100 worth of the newly introduced 'Healthy Herbal Skin Lotion.' We will also include some 'value coupons' in the local newspapers to promote this initiative. These programs should help us to reach our sales targets.

"I believe this will pave the way for a smooth transition to our exciting new line of cosmetics planned for introduction in 2025."

Reordering Priorities

Our reluctance or inability to make a clean break with an entrenched lifestyle is one of the main reasons why people get 'bored' or feel 'trapped' in an old routine. Here are two examples to demonstrate how a firm resolve to change one's priorities can solve this problem.

I) Generating Funds for a Long-Postponed Vacation:
Ralph and Karen are seriously considering a summer vacation in Rome, the Eternal City, which they have been dreaming about for many years. Their good friends, the Rawlings, have invited them for an extended holiday. The problem is that they have not been able to save enough money for the trip all these years. They estimate that the total out-of-pocket expenses would come to about $6,000, of which only $2,000 is in their holiday fund.

After a great deal of discussion and soul-searching, they have come up with a realistic plan that necessitates a rearrangement of their current spending priorities. Here is how it goes:

(a) Cut down our twice-monthly golf, to save $100. This will free up $600 within the next six months.
(b) Redirect the annual bonus of $1,000 (which was earlier earmarked for new furniture—this can wait for another year).
(c) Sell some pieces of little-used jewelry, currently sitting idly in the bank vault, expected to generate about $1,500.
(d) Cancel subscriptions for six magazines, their athletic club membership and wine club delivery—a combined saving of $1200.

Tallying up these austerity measures, they were pleasantly surprised to discover that the projected budget gap of $4,000 for the Roman Holiday can easily be met. They enthusiastically embraced this new priority plan.

II) Resolving Family Disputes:
Bob, a gentle, kind-hearted, and spiritually oriented individual, is bothered by an erstwhile disagreement with Jason, his brother-in-law. The dispute centers around the appropriate distribution of an inheritance among family members. Bob wants to put this vexing issue behind him. He is more interested in restoring his peace of mind: not accumulating property. He doesn't mind accepting a smaller share of the inheritance for himself, so that he can move on with his life. He also values family solidarity and wants to reestablish good personal relationships. He is eager to settle the dispute amicably, before next Christmas. He has decided to call Jason and offer a compromise plan. He figures that this generous initiative will be welcomed by Jason.

III) Clearing Household Clutter:
Here is a final example that will strike a sympathetic chord with readers who may have been procrastinating certain unpleasant but necessary tasks.

The Wilson family knows that their garage is messy and cluttered; it has been this way for a long time. So much junk has been stored there with the result that there is no room to move around, let alone park their car. They have been meaning to clean, repaint and spruce up the place for several months but never got around to doing so. Here is their priority plan:

"We are going to hold a garage sale during the President's Day weekend. Leaflets will be distributed in our neighborhood, one week before the event. Arrangements have been made to put an ad in the local paper.

Whatever stored stuff doesn't sell will be donated to the Salvation Army. In that event, we may be able to take a 'tax write-off' as per the advice of our accountant. We are also planning to buy a new car and will be able to keep it parked in the garage, instead of the curb.

"We are excited about the prospect of getting rid of many unwanted items and using the sales proceeds as a down payment on the new car."

Chapter Summary

There are some important lessons emerging from these case studies:

There comes a time in life when you realize that you need to try a different approach to solve a long-standing problem. You are convinced that the status quo is no longer acceptable. Or perhaps it doesn't pay to continue with that old strategy due to new resource constraints, changing priorities, altered family circumstances, or failing health. You have concluded that staying on the present path would be a waste of time and money. You say to yourself: "Perhaps the best solution would be to consider an altogether different strategy, even though it could be risky. It is time to shift gears."

1. Every decision must be accompanied by an appropriate strategy to accomplish the stated goal. The 'decision environment,' coupled with the availability of resources and willingness to accept trade-offs, determines the appropriate implementation strategy.
2. The chosen solution must fit the problem. Otherwise, it can backfire. This may sound obvious but is often forgotten.
3. One must scout for and find appropriate substitutes to fill existing 'resource gaps.' Without a clear, viable plan to do so, the decision can become empty of 'fuel.'

4. Similarly, when a preferred resource becomes too expensive, try to find a cheaper alternative. This requires both creativity and imagination.

5. Re-ordering of priorities can, in most cases, help to take care of changing economic circumstances. Those who are willing and able to make the requisite lifestyle adjustments can have a smooth transition from one stage to the next.

6. Make judicious use of appropriate incentives/disincentives (carrots and sticks) to influence human behavior. This strategy should help to secure the cooperation of others who are needed to implement your decisions.

7. Let the principle of 'comparative advantage' be your guide to allocate resources as efficiently as possible. This means:

    (a) Concentrate on doing those few tasks in which you excel, leaving everything else to others.

    (b) Decide on the appropriate division of labor among members of the household, based on their respective talents and interests, rather than some preconceived notion of traditional chores.

    (c) Make use of all available outsourcing opportunities, wherever and whenever possible, to free up time and energy. This should help to reduce stress and restore the much-valued 'work-life-balance' sought by many harried working parents.

8. Try to anticipate future financial needs and save regularly and consistently for potential large expenses such as (a) children's education, (b) emergency/rainy-day fund, (c) vacation/travel, (d) purchase of major appliances, and (e) retirement. This is the

single most important step you can take to promote lifelong financial security.

9. Be willing to compromise, concede and negotiate with others (whenever feasible) to resolve lingering conflicts.

10. Ignore 'sunk costs.' There isn't much you can do to undo past actions that misfired. Instead, try to take advantage of emerging opportunities to redirect resources intelligently.

Chapter VI
Overcoming Hurdles & Seeking Success

The Eagle Paradigm: A Useful Lesson from the Natural World

The animal kingdom provides many excellent examples demonstrating how they go about making effective decisions. Consider how an eagle hunts its prey. We homo-sapiens can learn a great deal from studying its behavior.

a) The Triggering Mechanism:
    Driven by the pangs of hunger and the need to feed its off-spring, the eagle decides to spring into action. It must hunt or else starve!

b) Strong Motivation:
    Hunger and the imperative to provide for its young growing family constitute a very compelling and urgent motive to act. The constant cries from the starving chicks can't go ignored.

c) Strength of Purpose:
    Action is urgently needed. It cannot be put off for a more convenient time. The eagle instinctively knows: "It is now or never."

d) Need for Careful Planning:
   The eagle must pick a suitable prey within a convenient striking distance. The closer the target, the better. If no prey is
   within sight, the hunter must be willing to go as far as it
   takes to scout and find suitable prey.

e) Timing:
   She needs to calculate the most opportune time to pounce on
   her prey: the element of surprise is critical—otherwise the prey
   will escape. The whole effort can then end in failure.

f) Resources Needed:
   Time: Patiently watching for a suitable prey to be sighted is a
   prerequisite for springing into action. This may take a long time.
   After assessing the likely distance where the prey is located, she
   must calculate (estimate) how long it will take to fly there. Does
   she possess the requisite agility and speed?

g) Energy: A lot of physical strength and energy are needed to
   pounce, pick up, carry the prey, and fly back to the nest. Even
   more so, if it is too heavy. She must also patiently feed the chicks
   before having her own dinner.

h) Skills: Coordination of various hunting faculties is critical for
   success. Ability to sight a suitable prey, fly there quickly, pounce
   upon and pick it up before it escapes, and bring it home in tact,
   require speed and dexterity.

i) Execution: After the prey is sighted and caught, she must haul it away to her nest as quickly as possible. The mission becomes a success only after this task is accomplished.

j) Potential Risks: Every hunting expedition the eagle undertakes is fraught with risks. The prey may try to escape, sensing potential danger. Some other predators may snatch it away before she gets into the act. The prey might be too big or too heavy (a bad miscalculation) to be carried back safely. It could fall down from her talons enroute. Or perhaps, it might be too small, not worth all the effort expended on the hunt! Sometimes the entire mission may have to be aborted midstream—due to bad weather.

There is the ever-present risk of disappointment and failure. But that possibility is not going to deter the eagle from trying again and again until she succeeds. She knows that 'learning by doing' never stops. If she fails the first, second or even a third time, those failures provide valuable lessons (a la experience) for future expeditions.

Summary: Successful hunting requires many innate (as well as acquired) skills. She must put together all the necessary parts in the right balance:

Timing (patiently waiting for the best moment to strike) +
Scouting and locating a suitable prey +
Agility (adequate flying speed) +
Energy (strength to circle around and fly over long distances) +
Confidence in her ability to get the job done +
Hunting experience (required to get ahead of rivals).

Concluding Remarks: Undoubtedly the eagle is a consummate master at making effective decisions: from conception to planning, preparation, execution and harvesting the results. This entails:

Knowing exactly what she wants: Her goal is to feed the hungry chicks waiting in the nest and herself (in that order).

Searching for a viable solution: watching, waiting, scouting, surveying the field and looking for a suitable prey.

Weighing all available options: Wondering which potential prey to go after—assuming there are a few available prospects within striking distance.

Doing a quick cost-benefit calculation: Is it better to go after a small, sluggish prey available nearby or a larger one farther away? What is the probability of a successful hunt?

Selecting the best available option: Go for the quick kill.

Implementing the decision: Take off, fly, pounce on the prey, pick it up, fly back, and feed the chicks.

Mission accomplished!

Conflicts

Here is a quote:

"The presence of conflicting forces or impulses within a single mind is a normal experience and the mind itself may not be fully aware of all the contending forces it is harboring" (Christopher F. Chabris: The Stranger Within).

"While the emotional part of your mind wants to indulge, the rational part warns: 'Don't do it; it is not for you, and you will regret it later.'"

This is a classic case of your senses urging you to succumb to a temptation or indulge in what you consider to be an immoral/unethical act. At the same time, your better judgment counsels you to defer or forego immediate gratification. The push and pull of these opposite forces leave you confused. You now face a dilemma or quandary.

A dilemma is defined as a situation requiring a choice between equally desirable/undesirable activities. A quandary is 'a state of perplexity or uncertainty, especially as to what to do.'

Such situations can give rise to many psychological difficulties, viz:

a) It becomes hard to evaluate the benefits and costs of the action in an objective, dispassionate manner.

(b) Available choices (options) are equally desirable/undesirable and there is no clear winner.

(c) There is an underlying ethical problem: regardless of what you do, you may regret your choice later.

(d) Your priorities are not clear-cut, resulting in confusion about which action is desirable at first.

(e) Fear of what could happen, regardless of whichever alternative you pick.

(f) A panic attack, wishing you did not have to face the situation.

(g) You wish you could postpone the decision or push away the problem being faced.

Here are two classic case studies illustrating the situation:

(1) In The Odyssey, Homer describes how the hero, knowing how the irresistible lure of the enchanting songs of the sirens would force him to their fold and end up endangering his mission, orders his crew to tie him to the ship's mast. He tells them not to relent and free him even if he begs them to do so. He knows he cannot resist the siren's call. His avowed desire to complete the voyage and return home to be united

with his family comes into direct conflict with the temptation posed by the sirens. Using this Commitment Strategy, he resolves the conflict between a strong emotional temptation and the avowed goal of completing his historic voyage and uniting with his family.

There are few parallels in classical literature depicting how the tussle between an irresistible emotional pull comes into conflict with one's long-term goals, threatening to sabotage the whole edifice.

Here is how Odysseus resolves the dilemma:

1. I know I will fall victim to the siren's haunting music, preventing me from continuing my voyage.
2. Therefore I must act proactively and take steps to avoid falling into their trap.
3. I do not want to be sidetracked into doing something which I know I will regret later.
4. I will make it impossible for me to succumb to this short-term temptation by asking my crew to tie me up to the ship's mast.
5. I have instructed them not to listen to my pleas to free me even if I beg them to do so when I am lured by the sirens. To ensure that this strategy works, I will get them drunk and put wax in their ears!
6. This plan will ensure that we can sail past the sirens, ignoring their songs, and win the ultimate prize of reaching our goal.

Here is a modern version of how to implement a commitment strategy:

Once you commit yourself to a certain course of action and device a suitable strategy to reach that predetermined goal, you can avoid being sidetracked by other short-term temptations/distractions. To ensure that you carry out your commitment faithfully and enhance the likelihood of success, some psychologists recommend that you openly declare your intentions (plan of action) to a trusted friend who can 'enforce' the commitment you made to yourself. If you fail to follow through, you agree to donate a predetermined sum of money to a charity that you hate! Or spend it on something you totally dislike— as a form of punishment.

Here is another classic example of a 'conflicted mind':

In Shakespeare's celebrated play, Hamlet is a tragic figure conflicted by the thought "To be or not to be—that is the question." He is torn between the desire to avenge his father's murder at the hands of his treacherous Uncle Claudius—and his strong belief that killing Claudius while the latter is engaged in prayer would send him to Heaven (rather than Hell, where he belongs). Hamlet is indecisive: he does not want Claudius to go to Heaven because that would be a reward rather than punishment for the perpetrator of a heinous crime.

Unlike Odysseus, Hamlet's inability to resolve the conflict between two powerful forces—his emotional need to seek vengeance and his reluctance to admit the possibility that Claudius might end up in Heaven—leaves him in a quandary.

The Nature of Conflicts in General

Conflicts are often internally generated tensions within your mind. They are the result of a simmering tug-of-war between the possibility of 'unconstrained action' and the reality of many constraints that inhibit your freedom to do what you want. One way to look at this problem is to imagine this tug-of-war as a clash between what is expedient and what is ethical.

Such conflicts arise when a particular "desire, interest, action, activity or event is incompatible with another of equal merit."

For those who have difficulty ordering their priorities, the underlying conflicts create a situation where decision paralysis ensues. Until you carefully think through and sort out the available options and accept one of them, you will be stuck in limbo. Here are some examples:

1. Extra Income or Family Time Together?

Ralph needs to work overtime, at least eight hours per week, to supplement his income to be able to meet the family's current lifestyle. If he does this, the time spent playing with his children during evenings and weekends, which they enjoy immensely, must be sacrificed. He is conflicted between these competing objectives: Should he earn more income to pay those recurring bills, which requires sacrificing precious family time together, OR forget overtime altogether and accept a lower standard of living? He is wondering what to do.

A similar problem was being faced by Joe, a department store manager. Joe was distressed that he was not earning a sufficiently high income to pay for summer camps, dancing and music lessons and other extracurricular activities for his teenage children. He knew that most youngsters in his social circle took part in such enrichment programs. He doted on his children, spending several hours each week playing games, fishing, taking them to various sports events and other cultural pursuits. Without consulting his family, he decided to work 'overtime' to earn extra income to pay for those 'enrichment programs,' which resulted in his not having any fun-time with the kids. The youngsters were not informed about their dad's decision. They missed their fun-time with him and became withdrawn and resentful. When Joe realized how miserable the kids were, he decided to go back to his former routine, gave up overtime work and resumed their former relaxed lifestyle.

2. Interpersonal Conflicts

Disagreements/differences of opinion, leading to perpetual arguments among individuals (spouses, siblings, friends, parents/children, employer/ employee, etc.), is a common phenomenon. There is often an underlying psychological warfare going on—which may be hidden or out-in-the-open that creates tension and stress, resulting in ruptured relationships. These center around:

1. Financial issues, such as (a) who gets to decide how to spend family income, (b) the relative importance of different categories of expenditures, and (c) allocation of current income between present and future needs.
2. The appropriate division of labor—especially household chores—among family members.
3. Degree of personal life satisfaction (quality of life) derived from one's professional work vs. family life is often a bone of contention between spouses. Arguments about the so-called 'work-life-balance'—especially about the need for additional current income to satisfy material aspects of life vis-à-vis availability of leisure time to pursue other cultural/family 'fun' activities.
4. Divergent views about the necessity/importance of close personal relationships with extended family members.
5. Ownership disputes about various assets and liabilities. Should assets/liabilities be designated separately as 'his,' 'hers,' 'ours,' or all 'jointly owned'?

6. Affinity toward different lifestyles based on one's upbringing, tastes, preferences as well as divergent philosophical and cultural values. Such divergent views are manifested in the degree of importance one attaches to social life, obligations to members of the extended family and shared interests regarding literature, art, music, travel, sports, etc.

There is often a fundamental disagreement among spouses or (one's better half) about the relative importance of these matters. Often people are not ready to give up what they consider personally fulfilling to them. Rather than allowing these disagreements to create constant tension and discord, the couple can try to reach a workable compromise by meeting each other's needs 'halfway.'

The Importance of Compromise

1. The meaning of compromise:
There are two types of compromise, a solution to resolve an existing conflict.

The first involves self: It is a recognition of the necessity to give up, alter or modify one's existing 'values, beliefs or habits' to achieve some worthy goal. In other words, you must be prepared to make an accommodation (concession or sacrifice) of some sort so that you can deal with an internal conflict. This happens when you are forced to change your behavior (say reduce or eliminate intake of sweets—which you enjoy) to achieve healthier outcomes—to lower blood sugar levels due to diabetes.

The second type involves a partial willingness to accept or appreciate another person's point of view or position on an important issue you were hitherto unwilling to appreciate.

2. The need to compromise arises:

When opponents realize that they cannot find a workable solution to a vexing problem unless and until each party is willing to alter, modify, concede, or make some adjustment to their existing position/point of view. The essence of a compromise is to find a 'middle path' or a 'workable solution,' which helps to reduce tension and move toward a mutually agreeable formula, satisfactory to all.

3. The nature of compromise:

A compromise can only arise when the disputants realize that it is in their mutual interest to find a middle ground (or workable solution) rather than hold on to the current 'uncompromising' standoff. The 'standoff' may have gone on for a prolonged period, resulting in continued mental strain, discomfort, or damage to their relationship. Therefore, each party becomes ready and willing to find some common ground to soften their respective positions and work toward finding a mutually agreeable solution or compromise.

4. When to compromise:

Obviously, the decision to compromise can happen only when the disputants realize that softening their current untenable positions (disagreements) will improve their overall long-term wellbeing. The concessions each party is willing to make will determine how the compromise works out.

5. How much to compromise:

This depends on how dogmatic and recalcitrant the opponents are, which has kept them apart. The degree of flexibility they evince will depend on their perception of the potential gains from making some concessions. Each will expect the opponent to concede as much as possible, while trying to minimize the concessions they are willing to make. How the disagreement between the parties is resolved depends on who is more interested (or desperate) to find a workable solution. There will be a 'power struggle' to determine how much more one can gain at the expense of the other, eventually leading to a compromise, benefitting both parties.

Benefits & Costs of Compromising

Compromise takes place because you realize that it is in your long-term interest to make some concessions or sacrifices to achieve what you desperately want. The psychic/financial costs of giving up or conceding your position to secure a solution (which has hitherto eluded you) should be less than the potential benefits you expect from such an agreement. Otherwise, you would not be willing to compromise. Each party will be better off when the perceived compromise-solution costs them less than the resulting flow of benefits. This results in a 'win-win' situation, benefitting everyone.

Decision-making and the Art of Compromise

Conflicts and disagreements between people arise from stark differences in personal priorities, values, firmly held beliefs or entrenched habits. Such personality differences often lead to interpersonal strife, tension and intolerance for the other party's position or point of view.

Unfortunately, when this happens between spouses, siblings, friends, neighbors, or colleagues, it can cause a great deal of pain and suffering. One possible remedy is to find some type of compromise—which can defuse the tension. When the feuding parties come to realize that the advantages and benefits of such compromise makes it eminently desirable and timely, steps can be taken to bring about a reconciliation. This will pave the way to seek and find a mutually agreeable solution, a decision which can benefit everyone concerned.

More on Conflict Resolution & Compromise

Since lingering, unresolved conflicts can wreak havoc by robbing your peace of mind, it is wise to resolve them as quickly as possible. This helps to regain mental equanimity and restore harmonious relationships.

When people hold different points of view or opinions on a given subject and are unable or unwilling to find common ground, it leads to disagreements and can eventually lead to 'conflict.' Failure to concede, compromise or find mutually agreeable solutions to the conflict can result in either "Let us agree to disagree" or permanent estrangement. When this happens between spouses/couples/companions, family life can become stressful and can lead to mutual recrimination.

This can sometimes become a difficult problem to solve as family chores multiply, especially with the advent of children. Childcare and other umpteen, ever-increasing list of tasks associated with modern family life consumes a lot of time and energy. Especially with two-income families, both spouses being engaged in their respective duties or lines of work, sharing family chores equitably can become a challenge.

When a couple decides to join in matrimony (or any other workable arrangement to share and care for each other), they can establish a list of tasks to be done by each, based on their respective skills and interests.

This list can form the basis of what each should do, subject to suitable adjustments and changes over time. This arrangement should form the basis for sharing family responsibilities.

Here is a workable strategy to assign everyday household tasks.

(1) Determine who has the comparative advantage in doing a particular task (based on experience, abilities, expertise, and interests).
(2) Determine how much time, energy (effort) and skills are needed to perform major task categories.
(3) Assign different group of tasks to each person—on a temporary or experimental basis and see how this works out.
(4) If there are tasks which both must do together and share equally to accomplish as a team, draw up that list.
(5) Determine tasks that can be 'outsourced'—which neither spouse wants to or is willing to do.
(6) These lists can be called 'Mine,' 'Yours,' 'Ours,' and the rest 'Outsourceable.'

If this system works reasonably at first and later needs tinkering/adjustments, such changes can be made from time to time.

A similar give-and-take approach to resolve disagreements about (1) household spending priorities, (2) investing for retirement, (3) vacation planning, (4) child rearing, and (5) religious/cultural activities, etc., should help to bridge the gaps that are commonly observed to exist between spouses.

All too often, each party comes to the union with divergent philosophies, values and habits inculcated while they were growing up. Sometimes these attitudes can become 'diehard'—each party adhering to their pet point of view, thinking theirs is somehow superior to the views held by the other. In turn, such entrenched positions become a fertile ground for 'in-fighting' and unwillingness to compromise.

To reduce the resulting marital friction, promote harmony and secure peace of mind, one must be willing to listen carefully to the other party's point of view. Areas of disagreements can then be negotiated amicably. This requires a sincere desire to compromise. Giving each other some room for individual decision-making, while upholding the paramount need for the family's long-term wellbeing and quality of life, can work wonders. When each person recognizes that the other party's cooperation and happiness is key to their own, previous disagreements can disappear like fog in the sunshine!

We should acknowledge that each one of us is a bundle of strengths and weaknesses as well as positive and negative personality traits. Recognizing this fact is the key to fruitful negotiation and workable compromises.

Mistakes

The term 'mistake,' when applied to decision-making, can have varying interpretations. There are different ways in which the term can be understood, depending on which point of view fits a particular situation.

As stated earlier, people think of a decision as a 'mistake' when you failed to achieve the expected results. This could be the result of any number of reasons. Perhaps the decision was premature, ill-considered and ill-timed—popularly termed 'too little or too late.' Perhaps the decision was based on inadequate, outdated, or misleading information. Or it was not the right solution to the problem you were facing. The decision was made without analyzing all its potential costs and consequences or not carried out or monitored properly. It was arrived at hastily and failed to anticipate some negative externalities which later became a big liability. Or it was impulsive, made under duress, executed haphazardly, and doomed to failure.

What all this means is that the decision failed to deliver the intended positive results. In addition, it created additional difficulties (or new headaches) which now must be dealt with.

A second way to interpret a mistake is to ask whether the decision infringed on prevailing standards of morality, ethical norms, or legal constraints. Sometimes people tend to forget or even ignore such lofty considerations. In the quest for quick short-term rewards, notions of what is immoral, unethical, or illegal are brushed aside. Later, one may feel the pangs of conscience and repent such transgressions—a belated recognition that the decision was a 'mistake.' Such cases are all too common in certain competitive games, sporting events and investment schemes (such as the Ponzi Pyramid Scheme). Regardless of the individual's underlying motivation or rationale to participate in them, it is a 'zero sum game' because the benefits enjoyed by one party are derived at the expense of others. Sometimes these personal choices end up having many anti-social consequences (negative externalities), as when people engage in actions that adversely affect the environment or the wellbeing of fellow citizens.

This may well be unintentional or done without considering their adverse impact on third parties. Unabashed selfishness, greed, willful negligence, and the single-minded aim of minimizing personal cost or inconvenience to oneself, lead some people to shift the costs of their actions on to others—forcing society to shoulder the resulting burdens.

This is all too common with economic crimes such as theft, arson, burglary, environmental pollution, etc., or other non-economic indulgences such as careless disposal of waste products, drunken driving, and uncivil behavior in general.

Probably there is no one who has not made one kind of decision mistake or another. Despite all your hard work, sincerity, attention to detail, wisdom and experience, some decisions turn out to be mistakes—in hindsight.

Note that all mistakes are recognized as such only in retrospect—presumably, no one admits to making a mistaken decision (knowingly or intentionally) beforehand!

Sometimes a family member, friend, trusted advisor, or other well-wisher may think of your impending decision as a mistake and even point out why that may be so (in their opinion). You may be persuaded to heed their counsel and re-think the decision, or you may still go ahead with your plans regardless of their warnings—only time will tell whether it was the right thing to do!

In summary: However ill-conceived a decision may be, no one will willingly admit that it was a 'mistake' ex-ante. However, some folks will reluctantly admit that decisions that did not pan out were probably mistakes: ex-post!

Why do mistakes happen in the first place?

There are umpteen causes, reasons, and explanations, depending on the type of decision involved and the context in which it takes place. We can place them into two broad categories:

Omission and Commission:

Acts of Omission happen when you fail to do something which is required, necessary, mandatory, or important to preserve, protect and ensure your future health, safety, and wellbeing.

Omissions could be the result of ignorance, neglect, laziness, inertia, or a general lack of resources. Failure to act properly at the right time (proactively) is a common phenomenon.

This only becomes apparent when the adverse consequences of inaction begin to emerge gradually. You realize, belatedly: "I should have known, acted, and taken steps to deal with it then. I missed the opportunity, messed up, did not pay attention, was negligent, irresponsible/lax" and similar profuse expressions of regret.

To elaborate: although no deliberate, conscious decision was involved, the mere omission or failure to act is deemed a 'mistake.' Here are some examples:

1. I failed to accumulate sufficient funds for our retirement. I got caught up with too many other pressing financial obligations.
2. I should have bought 'flood insurance' on the property; the storm flooded my basement; now I must face huge repair bills.
3. I failed to obey the posted speed limits; I was driving absent-mindedly and ended up with a court summons for willful negligence.
4. I forgot (neglected) to file my income tax returns in time; now I must pay a huge penalty with accumulated interest on back taxes.
5. I made a big mistake ignoring my doctor's warnings about kidney failure resulting from excessive alcohol consumption; if I

had listened to her warnings, I wouldn't be desperately looking for a kidney transplant now.

6. I wish I had heeded my mother's plea to stop gambling; she had warned me repeatedly how it would eventually lead to my financial ruin.

7. Not heeding my lawyer's advice to settle the lawsuit earlier was a big mistake; the Court's final verdict has now cost me twice as much.

8. If we had done periodic maintenance on the heating system, it wouldn't have conked out unexpectedly in the middle of winter leaving us without heat for many days.

Acts of Commission, on the other hand, are the offspring of decisions stemming from poor judgment, over-confidence, ego-centric acts, impulsive spending, emotional outbursts, and other manifestations of lack of self-control.

Here is a sprinkling of examples from my own life—these have taught me invaluable lessons and insights about the formidable power of decisions to shape our lives—for better or worse!

1. Over-confidence: I invested a considerable sum of money in some technology stocks pretending I knew how to make a fortune by anticipating the future. Alas, much to my chagrin, my confidence was misplaced, and I managed to lose a good deal of money.

2. Misplaced Trust: I loaned a substantial amount of my savings to a colleague who was facing hard times and who I thought was honest and trustworthy; it was a classic case of poor judgment.

3. "Have it; but don't need it/Need it, but don't have it" On several occasions, I took my umbrella on my neighborhood walks thinking that the rain was imminent; but the sun shone brightly. At other times, when I convinced myself that carrying the umbrella might be unnecessary, the clouds burst, drenching me profusely, proving me wrong again.

4. Giving Unsolicited Advice: I was trying to make a convincing argument to persuade my friend from taking a certain foreign trip (because of the possibility of terrorism in that country). She still went ahead with her plans, ignoring my warnings. She thoroughly enjoyed the trip, much to my great relief.

5. Hard work doesn't always payoff: I bought a new automobile after thorough and painstaking research. It still turned out to be a 'lemon' costing me a great deal of financial and emotional distress. I ended up wasting a lot of time visiting the dealership's repair shops.

6. Failure to own up: Here is an example of behavior I am not proud of: I used to take money from my grandmother's saving kitty when I was an adolescent, to indulge my taste for cookies and chocolates. Upon being discovered, I denied having done so. Rather than condemning my clandestine behavior, she then lovingly told me why I should be forthcoming and truthful. Her painstaking instruction taught me an invaluable lesson: when you make a mistake, admit it, try to learn from it, and be thankful that it gave you an opportunity to become smarter and wiser.

7. Knowledge is Power: Frugality, it seems, can sometimes be carried to excess! I used to walk to school to save the bus fare; I then ended up with a bad headache and sore feet, jeopardizing

my health. Knowing which particular resource one should try to economize at any given time is critical to our physical and mental wellbeing.

8. To summarize: Looking back and reflecting on the lessons I learnt: 'While hindsight is almost always perfect, it doesn't help you (one bit) to avoid past mistakes. Foresight is priceless but seldom available when you need it most.' Painful experiences and losses taught me how to be a better decision-maker.

Regrets

Of all the phrases that express one's nostalgic feelings for certain past events, none is more poignant than "It might have been." When this is specifically applied to decisions, the word 'regret' comes to the fore—as in (1) "I should have done it but failed to act" and (2) "I shouldn't have done it but did it anyway." The first signifies a belated recognition of 'missed opportunities' that were once available to you and should have been seized—but were let go. The second refers to rash decisions made earlier that seemed appropriate then but were mistakes—with the benefit of hindsight. The saying 'If youth knew and old age could' aptly sums up these divergent situations.

How does this happen often and why?

Our attitudes, beliefs, habits, opinions, and worldview (philosophy of life) undergo changes during the lifecycle. Although we inhabit the same body from birth to death, the mind (consisting of umpteen experiences, observations, accumulation of knowledge and reflective wisdom) provides us with a wider perspective and understanding of the hidden mysteries of life. As a result, some of the choices made earlier may now appear undesirable or unsound while 'The Road Not Taken' seems to have been full of promise. How you evaluated those choices partly determined the degree of satisfaction you derived from them. You learnt to use your wisdom, training, mental faculties, and judgment to make the choice that best fitted your needs and circumstances. Only time could tell whether your choices met your expectations and how satisfied you were with them. To paraphrase the Roman Emperor-Philosopher Marcus Aurelius: "Your life is what your decisions/choices make it."

Whenever those choices did not work out as expected or disappointed you, regrets came to haunt you. This too is an unavoidable and normal part of everyone's life experiences. They may be thought of as periodic acts of cleansing. They help to let go of things that were beyond your control. All you can do now is learn to relax, reflect calmly and make befitting decisions in the future that will leave you more satisfied.

The Blame Game

As we have seen, regardless of how earnestly and carefully you try to make decisions, some mistakes will inevitably creep up 'after the fact.' Or the results may fall short of initial expectations, leaving you disappointed, frustrated and unsatisfied.

When this happens, you have three possible choices.

1. Accept the outcome without complaint. You know that many factors can intervene between a decision (made in the present) and its coming to fruition (later in the future). These are beyond your control.

2. Revisit the decision carefully and as objectively as possible. Try to find out why it failed to deliver. This process may reveal valuable information and insights which can help you to make better decisions in the future; this becomes a learning experience.

3. Shift the 'blame' for under-performance to somebody else, absolving yourself of responsibility for the subpar results. (This may give you short-term satisfaction but does not solve the underlying problem.) This step is 'comforting' but treacherous. It prevents you from taking full and complete responsibility for your actions and loses the opportunity to learn from the mistakes you have made. It assumes that you took the right course of action, that you knew exactly what to do and executed your decision faultlessly. Since the outcomes were disappointing, some other person or agent is held responsible for under-performance.

There are many possible explanations for this behavior pattern.

a. The subject assumes that their actions were perfect, faultless, and beyond reproach. They did everything possible to 'do the right thing'; therefore, the expected positive outcomes should have followed in tandem. When this failed to materialize, they assume that 'some powerful spirit' must have intervened to deny them their well-deserved success.

b. The outcome was brought about by some other external agent (such as your boss or coworker) who failed to reward you appropriately for your efforts. For example:

If you did not get a salary increase or bonus, your boss must be at fault for passing you over and favoring some other candidate.

Your poor 'grade' was the result of a test that included topics/questions that were not covered in the class or syllabus.

The credit card debts piling up were due to your spouse overspending the family budget.

You were late to arrive at the office for the meeting because of traffic jams, utterly beyond your control.

The job interview really went well; you were the most qualified candidate for the job, but the person finally selected happened to belong to a minority group (perhaps mandated by political considerations).

That investment was 'a sure bet' but an unexpected 'hostile takeover' did you in. No matter how much effort you put in, the game was rigged from the start; the chances of your winning were almost non-existent.

To summarize, some people habitually resort to engaging in the "Blame Game" to justify their actions, refusing to delve deeply into the real causes of their failures. By doing so, they deny themselves the opportunity to learn from their mistakes—often leading to a 'dead end.' To avoid this trap, it is best to keep an open mind and recognize that no one is infallible. Age, experience, hard work, intelligence, and wisdom do not always guarantee 'perfect results' while playing the game of life—there is always plenty of room to learn and improve.

Proverbs and Rules of Thumb

In every culture and geographic region of the world, earlier generations have gifted to posterity some of their thoughtful reflections on life. These are condensed in the form of proverbs.

These insights contain a great deal of wisdom, born of many hardships and lessons learnt while dealing with the many trials and tribulations of life. While some of these may have only limited appeal when applied to our own unique circumstances, others contain universal truths, worthy of recognition and adoption. It is up to you, dear reader, to pick and choose from this vast encyclopedia, some of which may appeal to you. They don't cost anything; are fun to read, review, put to use or discard as you seem fit. I provide below a sample of these gems for your consideration with appropriate footnote interpretations of my own.

"The journey of a thousand miles begins with the first step."

To meet difficult challenges, one must first begin the task, continue to make slow and steady progress and work toward ultimate success.

"Time and tide wait for none."

No one can ignore the laws of Nature. Be humble, no matter how important you think you are. If you wait for the perfect moment to start a project, you may be waiting for ever.

"Prevention is better than cure."

In every aspect of life, a great deal of resources can be saved by taking proactive/preventive action before some crisis hits. This is especially true of healthcare. A healthy lifestyle—consisting of a nutritious/wholesome diet, moderate daily exercise, annual medical checkups, adoption of safe driving habits and adequate sleep—can pay big dividends. Ignoring these sensible recommendations can result in expensive treatments, physical/psychic distress, and unnecessary suffering.

"If wishes were horses, beggars would ride them."

If you want something, you must be willing to put forth the requisite effort to get it; otherwise, it will remain an empty dream.

"He who knows the price of everything doesn't know the value of anything."

Prices are objective measures, ephemeral, and constantly fluctuate in response to the forces of supply and demand. The concept of 'value' is more permanent and personal, based on the important distinction between 'useful' and 'vital.'

"Would you abdicate choice in favor of chance?"

This is a question everyone must ponder and answer carefully. When you make decisions, you must be willing to take full responsibility for your choices. You must have the courage of your convictions and act prudently. Looking for excuses and selectively invoking 'bad luck' or blaming others for poor results is a sign of immaturity.

"You may have some of the things all of the time; many of the things some of the time, but not all of the things all of the time."

The unceasing quest for wanting everything, or "having it all," is pure chimera. This constant striving is a fool's paradise, setting you up for permanent disappointment. One should be willing and able to prioritize, select what is truly important and forego secondary things.

"When the going gets tough, the tough gets going."

Obstacles, failures, setbacks, disappointments, and losses are an integral part of life. The road ahead can be rough, hazardous, full of ups and downs, and even treacherous. If you are patient, persistent and determined to proceed to your destination, eventual success will ensue.

"A bird in hand is worth two in the bush."

For those who seek safety and security but dislike taking risk, it is better to accept a known small prize now rather than gamble for a bigger prize later.

"Yesterday is a cancelled check; tomorrow is a promissory note; today is ready cash; spend it wisely."

What has been done can rarely be undone. Hope springs eternal. The future is full of promise if you plan ahead by making good decisions today.

"Trust but verify."

If you are not sure about the integrity and trustworthiness of another party with whom you are going to do business, it is prudent to be skeptical and make sure that they are going to deliver what they promised.

Rules of Thumb

What are these? Where do they come from? Can they be depended upon?

Can a decision ever be reduced to a formula?

One can reasonably assume that some things that worked in the past—based on familiarity and repeated experience—can be expected to work again. 'You don't have to reinvent the wheel.'

Just as proverbs contain pearls of wisdom which can be used as guidelines for action, 'rules of thumb' can provide ready-made formulae for making decisions in certain situations. These are simple, straight-forward, and easy to follow—in most cases. Without detailed analysis, they can serve as tentative guidelines to help us move forward. You may think of them as 'no-brainer-recipes' or tentative guides to action.

Here are a few examples:

1. One should pay no more than 3.5 to 4 times' annual income for purchasing a house.

2. Potential lenders use the 28/36% rule when evaluating most mortgage loan applications: i.e.,

   28% of household income for monthly payment of principal, interest, and real estate taxes; and

   36% for all debt obligations.

3. Refinancing a mortgage is worthwhile if the new interest rate is at least 0.75% less than the current rate: alternatively, the reduced monthly payments should be sufficient to cover 'closing costs' of the new mortgage in about 24 months.

4. The percentage of income going toward instalment debt should be no more than 10%.

5. The proportion of retirement assets invested in stocks should be close to 120 minus your current age. (The logic behind this archaic formula is that you will have sufficient time to recover from stock market declines.)

6. Your emergency savings funds should cover three to six months' worth of monthly spending, depending on the stability of your job (cash flow).

7. Life insurance should equal ten times' annual salary to protect against accidental death.

8. The annual withdrawal rate of accumulated retirement funds should be no more than 4 to 5%, to provide for 20-25 years of retirement income.

9. One should try to save at least 10% of household income to provide for (1) retirement, (2) college education, (3) emergency funds, (4) vacation, and (5) replacement of household appliances.

10. Delaying Social Security benefits until age 70 can result in increased monthly payments of almost 8% for life —a very good 'rate of return,' indeed!

I Can't Make Up My Mind: What Should I Do?

'Make up your mind' is an exhortation commonly heard by those who have difficulty deciding. There could be many valid reasons for your unwillingness to commit to a certain course of action. The most common reason is the fear of adverse consequences. This fear springs from multiple causes such as:

i.   Lack of self-confidence.
ii. Fear of repeating previous mistakes: what if I make the same mistake again?
iii. Fear of criticism ("Why did you do that? You should have...")
iv. Confusion: The necessity of having to evaluate too many choices (which are baffling in their variety and complexity).
v.   Lacking clarity (not getting a good handle on what is really at stake).
vi. Inability to prioritize (everything seems equally important).
vii. Fear of rejection (What if I make the wrong move? Will the other person be agreeable to this request, suggestion, proposal, etc.?).

Coping Strategies:

1. Putting off the decision indefinitely.
   Comment: This is only a temporary solution. At some future time, you will have to resolve the problem. It makes sense to

think through all the pros and cons now and come up with a solution before the issue becomes even more difficult to tackle.

2. Wait for a signal from some benevolent extraneous source.
   Comment: This is a vain hope. Outside forces probably have no vested interest in your wellbeing.

3. Ask someone you trust who can give objective advice.
   Comment: This idea makes eminent sense. Observe how the advisor dissects the problem and comes up with the right solution (a great opportunity to learn from their example).

4. Delegate the task:
   Comment: Yes, this may work when you are overwhelmed with too many things to do. But will you be satisfied with whatever decision the delegate makes? Make sure the delegate knows your mind.

5. Toss a coin: Heads (Go for it); Tails (Don't do it).
   Comment: This may or may not work 50% of the time. Trusting your judgment is far better than trusting a coin's (non-existing) judgment.

6. Leave it to Nature:
   Comment: Mother Nature can only help those who are prepared to help themselves.

7. Hope the problem will eventually go away.
   Comment: It most probably will not—but could even get worse. Far better to address it now when you have some control over the situation.

Whatever be the cause of ambivalence, the only sensible solution is for you to make up your mind and act accordingly. Do your cost-benefit analysis carefully, trust your judgment and see what happens. There could be a steep learning curve: but eventually, success will follow.

Think of a baby learning to walk. At first, she falls frequently, gets hurt, and cries. Slowly and steadily, she learns the ropes. With every new baby step and encouragement from her mother, she becomes more confident of herself. She walks gingerly, falls, gets up, falls back, gets up again and this goes on repeatedly, many times. With persistent practice, she learns to gain balance, keeps moving, smiles, and finally gets the hang of it all! If learning by doing works for a child, it is true for adults as well.

If you have read this far, you know that no decision, however well-thought-out, can always deliver the outcomes you expect. This is true of expert decision-makers as well as novices.

Reasons Why Decisions Fail

"There is many a slip between the cup and the lip."

Regardless of how carefully and diligently you make decisions, they may fail to deliver the expected results. Or realized outcomes could fall short of expectations. If you were to analyze your past decisions, you might find something like the following (average results):

(a) 25%: Successful: Realized outcomes > = expected
(b) 25%: Satisfactory: Realized results = expected
(c) 10%: Disappointments: Realized < below expected
(d) 40% Failures: negative outcomes

Note: It might be a useful exercise to check your own experience in this regard.

A careful and objective review of your past performance should reveal many plausible reasons for the sub-optimal outcomes.

Obviously, it is not just the percentage of fruitful results (a + b) that you should look at: some decisions are far more consequential than others. Therefore, special attention should be given to those critical or weighty decisions that matter the most. Recall the previous classification (relative importance) of all decisions into three groups, i.e. (a) Routine = 80%; (b) Important = 15% and (c) Critical = 5%.

To improve the odds of getting what you want (in the future), it helps to be conscious of some of the common pitfalls (traps) that people knowingly or unknowingly fall into. Here are the most common culprits.

(I) Information Gap

Decisions based on spotty, outdated, insufficient or misleading information:

In our rapidly changing world, some facts and figures can become obsolete very fast. Financial decisions based on inaccurate prices, misquoted interest rates, outdated market surveys or unaudited numbers are a case in point. You may have observed that purveyors of statistical data/financial information frequently restate, alter, or modify previously published numbers. It is in your interest to verify and make sure that the information you rely on to make decisions is reasonably accurate and up to date.

(II) Laziness and Inertia

Even after making a well-considered decision, its implementation might be temporarily delayed. You might think that a little bit of delay does not matter much. Some other urgent problem might crop up, demanding redeployment of resources earmarked for the former project. This might even serve as a convenient excuse for delaying action! Or you may have 'second-guessed' yourself and intentionally put off the earlier decision. When timing is critical, a 'missed opportunity' can spell the difference between success and failure.

Does the phrase 'Too little, too late' ring a bell? 'Too little,' because the initial response was insufficient (in quantity or quality) to deal with the problem. 'Too late,' because failure to take timely action will necessitate additional outlays or extra effort. Initial hesitation, lack of clarity about your mission or prolonged delays in implementation are the usual culprits. Failure (inability) to meet your financial obligations is a case in point. A frequently neglected area is healthcare. Issues such as routine vision and dental care, oral hygiene, blood sugar control and inoculation against communicable diseases are often put in the 'backburner.' Later, when emergency situations force you to take urgent action, you wish you had taken care of these matters earlier when they were manageable, with fewer resources.

(III) Lack of Communication

At times, much to your dismay, the assumption 'Let George do it; it's his job' can be a big mistake. This often happens when the hypothetical 'George' fails to live up to his responsibilities, no matter how much you wish he had! It is possible that George is blissfully unaware of his role in carrying out your mission. Is he really a trustworthy, responsible person? Can he be expected to do what he is supposed to do? Is he interested in this delegated task at all? Without some reasonable assurance that George is willing to complete his part of the bargain, you may finally end up picking up the tab. To avoid this eventuality, there should be a viable plan/arrangement to seek George's explicit cooperation and compliance. Non-enforceable obligations have no legal standing and can come to haunt you later on.

(IV) Murphy's Law:
"If anything can go wrong, it probably will" is an abbreviated version of this remarkable proposition. Probably you have personally experienced the truth of this statement.

Moreover, Murphy's Law often seems to raise its ugly head at the most inconvenient, inopportune time and place. Airline flight cancellations or missed flights are a case in point. Have you ever encountered traffic jams and delays on your way to the airport? Or the car battery refusing to crank on a bitterly cold winter morning? A repairman not showing up for hours after the appointed time? A baby getting sick on a long holiday weekend, when her pediatrician is on vacation? A much-delayed insurance settlement check getting lost in the mail? Can't find an important tax record or warranty paper or bill of sale when you are desperately looking for them everywhere? Your laptop quits working just when you are in the midst of an important writing assignment?

The list goes on. Not much can be done about these mishaps—they just happen, validating Murphy's Law.

But it is possible to moderate the severity of the associated pain and inconvenience by having a proper back-up or substitute plan—the proverbial Plan B—and spare yourself much inconvenience.

It pays to be prepared. One can try to be proactive instead of being just reactive. The incidence of emergencies can be minimized by proper planning and preparation (wherever and whenever possible). To know how to overcome roadblocks, deal with setbacks and negotiate one's way through difficult situations takes planning, imagination, and wisdom.

(V) Depending on Blind Faith

Decisions based on untenable beliefs, superstitions, rumors, or misplaced trust can be detrimental to your physical, emotional, and financial wellbeing. Unfortunately, this happens all too often. Belief systems which held sway over previous generations may have lost their validity (and usefulness) today because of rapid changes in technology, political, social, and economic changes. Yet, bound by age-old traditions, many people are reluctant to part with them.

(VI) Superstitions:

The Random House Dictionary defines a superstition as "a belief or notion, not based on reason or knowledge, in or of the ominous significance of a particular thing, circumstance, occurrence, proceeding or the like. A system or collection of such beliefs."

By its very nature, a superstition belongs to a type of thinking known as "Post Hoc Ergo Propter Hoc," meaning 'After this, therefore because of this.' The hallmark of a superstition is its supposedly supernatural predictive power to influence an Event ' B,' unrelated to an Event 'A' which preceded it. Those who subscribe to some (untenable) age-old superstitions adhere to them (and defend their importance or validity) while others may find them hollow and devoid of meaning or substance.

Superstitions exert a profound influence on human behavior. They silently dictate what one can or cannot do. They may be specific to a religion, culture, geographic region, or ethnicity.

Here are some popular ones:

1. Certain letters of the alphabet are inauspicious while others are auspicious to name your child.
2. The # 4, 13, or (whatever you fancy) spell disaster and should be avoided.
3. Certain days of the week or hours of the day should be shunned—for marriage or new business ventures.
4. The presence (or absence) of certain animals, birds, noises (laughter, sneezing, etc.) are inauspicious. When you notice/hear them, do not venture outside.
5. Knocking on wood will keep 'evil spirits' away and protect you from harm.
6. Praying to or appeasing ancestral 'spirits' must precede buying or selling a house. The entrance to the house must face a certain direction—otherwise disaster will follow.

And the list goes on…

In short, the hallmark of a superstition is that a decision to carry out or desist from some activity or undertaking, is conditional on the presence or absence of a completely unrelated, extraneous signal or event.

In this way of thinking, success or failure of an undertaking is not based on the project's internal merits or demerits, but some other favorable or unfavorable signal emanating elsewhere.

It is not just simple activities of daily living that are the domain of superstitions: many important decisions pertaining to education, job/career, business, investments, marriage, child-rearing, housing, relocation,

199

retirement, etc., can be greatly influenced by them. In other words, they can hold sway over your entire life.

People tend to hold on to their superstitions wherever they go, unless and until they decide to discard them (selectively). Curiously enough, this may happen when they encounter non-superstitious people (who make decisions based on objective considerations alone) and realize how those earlier beliefs held them back or prevented them from exercising 'free will.'

Are you superstitious? Do you know anyone who is not? Have you had any meaningful discussions with others on this subject? Does some powerful superstition encourage or stand in the way of your making otherwise 'informed decisions'?

It is up to you to acknowledge the hidden power of those irrational beliefs, selectively discard those that don't make any sense, or continue to hold on to them—it is your choice!

(VII) **The Celebrity Syndrome** or following excessively opinionated advice. Note the key phrase 'excessively opinionated.' The newer term might be "Influencers." Those who render advice to others often think that their personal examples/achievements/experiences can be replicated or copied by others. "If I could do it, so can you" is the rallying cry. Being able to recognize the difference between well-meaning but ill-suited advice and its counterpart is critical.

Often there is a natural tendency to blindly imitate the example of people one admires (popularly known as 'hero worship'). Individuals who have achieved great success in different walks of life may serve as models for others, worthy of emulation. There could be much to admire and learn from their examples. However, you should be on guard before imitating them to save your own sanity. Why? Their unique backgrounds, circumstances, experiences, and degree of commitment to a cause could differ enormously from yours and mine. It would be a grave mistake to assume that what worked for a certain individual within a given context will also work for you. Although this should be self-evident, it is often assumed without question that there is a 'cookie-cutter' recipe for success. This is far from the truth.

(VIII) **Wishful Thinking:**

One should not harbor the illusion that there is a magic formula for success which can be applied universally. Although previous decisions of a certain kind may have paid off handsomely, the current environment may have turned hostile to them. This valuable lesson was brought to my attention by Krieger, an experienced citrus farmer. Here is what he said:

"Inadequate resources, diminished soil fertility and vastly different weather conditions stood in the way of repeating last year's bountiful orange harvest. This time around, the fruit needed more time to ripen because of paucity of sunshine during the critical final weeks before harvesting. The old pest control system was not as effective in warding off the new breed of bugs. Despite concerted efforts to salvage a good portion of my groves, I was unable to make a decent profit this year."

Sometimes you tend to make decisions without a fuller, clearer, deeper understanding of the degree of effort needed to achieve the stated goal. The inspiration or zeal with which you started the program is hard to sustain for a prolonged period unless you are deeply committed to it. While the spirit behind the decision may be laudable and sincere, the 'flesh is often weak' to sustain a high level of effort. Once the initial enthusiasm has passed, the true psychological cost of the program begins to take its toll—hammering away at one's determination and willpower. You must then make a momentous choice: do you stay committed to the goal or quit? This is the moment of truth—'crunch time,' as some prefer to call it—your sense of self-worth hangs in the balance.

A familiar example of this type of situation is what happens to New Year's Resolutions and other 'self-improvement' programs. The initial high-spirited enthusiasm is followed by inertia, inadequate follow-up, slow progress, tardiness, boredom and eventual dropping out. As everyone knows, it is easy to make promises (even to oneself!). You set yourself up for eventual disappointment when you discover that you cannot keep those promises. Is there a way out?

Yes! How about taking 'baby steps'—slow and steady at first, hardly noticeable, gradually stepping up the pace as you gain confidence (like all babies do when they begin to walk). Expectations of success must be toned down. They must be realistic, achievable, and spread over a long enough period. If springing like a rabbit doesn't cut it, why not adopt the proverbial 'snail's pace'? Or even imitate the sure and steady footsteps of the 'Patient Turtle' which is in no hurry to reach her destination?

One can learn a great deal from the animal world about effort, industry, patience, and perseverance.

Consider the industrious beaver—skillfully amassing twigs, tree branches and many other building materials to construct dams across streams and ponds.

Or the patient eagle, watchfully waiting for the right moment to pounce on its prey? Observe the forward-looking, hard-charging, goal-oriented squirrel—collecting acorns and nuts for the coming harsh winter.

Watch the humble penguin, strategically planning and picking the ideal spot to raise her chicks in an already crowded field.

Why not the persistent spider?

Of all the many valuable lessons a small insect can teach us, the legend of King Bruce of Scotland is both unique and heartening. Lying under a tree, despondent and weary after losing many battles with rebellious tribes and warlords, the King was pondering what to do next. He observed a spider weaving its web around a tiny branch in the nearby bush. Although the web being built was blown away repeatedly by the prevailing winds, the determined spider kept on building, not discouraged by its previous failures. Eventually, on the seventh try it succeeded in completing the web, settled down to rest, finally enjoying the fruits of its hard labor.

Observing how the spider managed to prevail against the powerful wind and build its nest, King Bruce thought to himself: "If a little insignificant insect can overcome such heavy odds, so can I. I will fight and win, no matter how long it takes."

Inspired by the example before him, Bruce got up, regrouped his battered army, rode on, managed to defeat his enemies, and regained his kingdom.

Example of a Winning Decision

When you are feeling very hungry, all you can think about is when, where and how soon you can find some food to take care of the pangs of hunger. If you can get the food quickly to satisfy that intense feeling of hunger, you will feel relieved and satisfied. If the food you actually get to consume turns out to be delicious and also satisfies your tastebuds, it is indeed a bonus—you not only feel well-fed, but also happy and contented.

Likewise, when you are confronted with a problem you need to find a viable solution so that it doesn't keep on nagging and distracting you for long. As often happens, finding a 'satisfactory' or workable solution does provide relief from vaunted stress but the decision may not provide any great sense of accomplishment. Occasionally, however, a well-thought-out decision can not only help solve the underlying problem, but its many (side) benefits can make you feel doubly happy and proud. This happens when the decision pre-empts new problems from raising their ugly head later, saving you precious resources.

Imagine a farmer whose farm is situated in a flood-prone area and consequently the crops are subjected to unpredictable, periodic flood damage. The farmer employs 'stop-gap' drainage measures to control floods as and when they occur, salvaging as much crops as possible. These measures are ad-hoc and their effectiveness is at best limited. They have not proved cost-effective in the past and the farmer has had a hard time dealing with this recurring problem.

Now suppose the farmer comes up with a permanent flood-control solution (a peripheral raised wall) which will keep the crops free from water damage. The farmer has done a thorough cost-benefit analysis and concluded that the project can be financially viable and rewarding. It will not only prevent floods from damaging the crops but also provide psychological relief from the recurring anxiety and financial losses created by unpredictable fluctuations in crop yields. If the project is implemented:

(1) It will ensure healthy and predictable future crop yields.
(2) Ensure a dependable steady cash flow.
(3) Saving on outlays for crop insurance (and cost of hedging).

(4) Freedom from mental anxiety about potential flood damage.

(5) Time and energy rendered free to devote to other matters.

Tough Decisions

Every now and then, you may run into situations where you wonder which option, among the ones available, is the most suitable one. Imagine reaching a fork in the road, during a dark night and you don't know which road will take you to your destination. You must guess (pre-GPS times!); there is no reliable information to go by. You must trust your instincts. Until you reach where you want to go, there is no telling if you took the right path. It is a 50/50 toss. What should you do?

One solution is to wait for a while, hoping that somebody will turn up and tell you what to do. But there is no guarantee that this will happen. And waiting at the fork could be a waste of precious time.

Or you take the plunge. Decide. Either you are right, or wrong. Only time will tell. Fortunately, many tough situations like this can be resolved with much less uncertainty. It is a matter of knowing the potential trade-offs, relative costs, possible future scenarios (outcomes), and resolving conflicts that still remain in the background.

Ask yourself (try to find out) what is the worst possible outcome for each available option. If one option seems more acceptable than another, then pick that option. If all of them are equally undesirable, then try to gather more information about their potential outcomes. This process should lead to greater clarity and eventually help you to make an acceptable option.

In some situations, all available options may seem equally bad or even hopeless. If that be the case, ask yourself: have I resolved internal conflicts lurking in the background? Do I fully understand the relative 'trade offs' I am now facing? If there is someone available who understands your predicament and whom you trust, perhaps they can help you to arrive at an acceptable solution. Or if there is still more time available to think it over, waiting a little longer can help.

When the final decision time arrives, since you have exhausted your time limit, make up your mind with all the courage you can muster and then wait for the results. Since you have done everything in your power to make the best possible decision, you can reconcile with whatever happens. The choice you made is now behind you; all you can do is to move forward.

Decisions by Default

There are many instances in life where you don't want to spend the time and effort needed to make a choice. You just want to minimize the energy involved in picking one among the many alternatives available. This is especially true when the choice in question is not important in your estimation. Or you may be pressed for time, feel bored or indifferent to the various choices being offered. You may be in a hurry to get on with whatever you are doing rather than agonize over this issue. You just want to pick something and move on. Such instances crop up all the time.

Let us look at some common examples.

1. Having to look through a long list of items in a restaurant menu, not knowing the real difference between those offerings.
2. Picking a particular flavor of ice cream among forty different varieties when you don't have a favorite, predetermined selection.

3. Choosing among different styles of color, shape, shade, or material in a tile showroom with hundreds of permutations/combinations from which to select.
4. Different settings in a computer's design/architecture.
5. Choosing a seat in a theater/airplane/public transport vehicle when you have no special preference.
6. Picking a 'payment plan' or 'investment choice' among those which are available—but difficult to comprehend or analyze.
7. A mind-boggling array of fashions/colors/shapes to choose from in a clothing store.
8. Telephone/internet/TV subscription plans which are confusing or hard to fathom or distinguish from one another.

And the list goes on…

In these situations, some people prefer to simply pick the 'default option,' which has been chosen by the service providers. Many establishments also make it easy for us to do business with them by suggesting:

'Today's Special,' at an unbeatable price.

'May we suggest an easy payment plan you can live with.'

"You do not have to do anything; simply sign on the dotted line."

"This offer will not be repeated again."

"Easy, convenient and …"

For many of us, the 'default decision' often eliminates the risk of picking a particular option which may later turn out to be unsatisfactory. Or sometimes hard to change—once you have made a choice of your own. The 'default option' is often simple, easy to understand or the least expensive. Or it may be the one which most people, without much expertise in the field might prefer. Especially when the plethora of available choices require special technical savvy to sort out!

Indeed the 'default option' is often an attractive way out for many of us. By opting for the 'easy way out,' you do not have to consider the pros and cons of every available option.

Undoubtedly there is an obvious convenience and simplicity to this arrangement.

However, there is a hidden downside to this way of making your choice. While 'default options' save us from considerable inconvenience for the moment, they may cost us a great deal in the long run.

Consider the following familiar examples.

a. You have chosen a gym/health club membership plan which continues indefinitely even when you do not use it. If you forget to cancel the membership before the automatic renewal date, you forfeit your deposit/periodic payment obligation.

b. You have opted to continue to charge your credit card automatically for various 'easy payment arrangements' such as magazine subscriptions, identity theft protection, unlimited credit report monitoring and credit score access, several types of recurring club dues, charitable donations, alumni events, sports activities, flight insurance plans and so on. Whether you use them or not, those automatic charges continue indefinitely if you do not review or cancel them in time. The convenience provided by the 'default option' can cost you a pretty penny. Indeed, many providers of these services count on your natural lethargy and inertia—or even take advantage of them—by providing such 'default options.' It is up to you, as always, to consider their costs and benefits.

c. People who have signed up for various employee benefit plans—such as automatic retirement contributions, some 401(k) plans, certain annuities, automatic saving schemes, etc.—are often unable or reluctant to examine all the available options. Many people simply check the "default option" without considering if it is suitable for their personal situation!

d. Another variation on the same theme is our natural reluctance to say "no." Consider the following common experiences most of you have had:

A Girl Scouts cadet approaches you with a basket of cookies to sell.

A teenager solicits a list of magazine subscriptions for the school athletic club.

A charity appeals through a telephone marathon requesting a donation to aid victims of domestic abuse.

The local Police Benevolent Association asks for your contribution to their Welfare Fund. At the supermarket's cash register, the cashier suggests that you put some money in their favorite fundraiser project.

You are asked to distribute pamphlets to your neighbors and friends seeking funds for Veterans.

Your colleagues ask for your participation in their favorite activities/sponsorships.

And the list goes on…

Moods and Decisions

Decisions are influenced by moods, feelings, and your current state of mind. Moods are subject to frequent changes, depending on your physical and mental health. You then see the world through 'rose-colored glasses,' distorting your perception. If you are undergoing extremes of pain, pleasure, sorrow or happiness, your judgment will lack objectivity.

Many external events like the weather, the behavior of people around you and your success or failure in dealing with them can influence how you feel and act. Powerful emotions can play havoc with your judgment. Feelings of sadness, anger, love, empathy, humility, and invincibility can profoundly affect one's normal response. When you are depressed or inebriated, your ability to think calmly and objectively is impaired.

Therefore, it is prudent not to make any important decisions under those circumstances. If any weighty issue comes up for consideration, you can wait until you feel 'normal' and in full control of your mental faculties. Or seek the opinion, input, or advice of a trusted person who can act on your behalf.

Another reason for deferring action is to avoid being coerced by eager and unscrupulous people who may want to take advantage of your vulnerabilities. Unfortunately, this experience is all too common. Watch out! Charlatans, opportunists, conmen, pious-looking 'pretenders' and their ilk are always scouting for innocent victims.

This is akin to deciding 'not to drive under the influence' or 'texting' while driving, two examples of sensible advance planning. Let someone else take control of the wheels temporarily while you relax after delegating your authority.

Procrastination

In our busy lives, when doing something is not considered urgent or important, it tends to be pushed aside for future consideration and action.

The difference between 'urgent' and 'important' tasks was explained earlier while discussing the 'Eisenhower Matrix.' It so happens that some things which are important are not necessarily urgent and vice versa. These twin attributes, importance and urgency, are not mutually exclusive. This distinction partly explains why we procrastinate.

Figure 9

Tasks

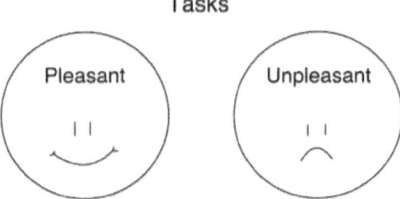

To fully explain this phenomenon, another useful distinction is called for: between pleasant and unpleasant tasks. These are, by their very nature, mutually exclusive.

Almost everyone likes to attend to all those pleasant, interesting, enjoyable tasks before taking up other essential but boring chores that compete for scarce resources (of time and energy).

Notice that while 'urgent' tasks must be dealt with almost immediately, many 'important' tasks can be put off indefinitely. Tasks that are both urgent and pleasant to carry out will get priority over those that happen to be urgent but unpleasant.For example, satisfying hunger is both urgent and pleasant. But filing your Tax Returns, especially as the deadline approaches, is urgent but unpleasant. Therefore, this task tends to be put off as long as possible. Some folks wait until the night of April 15 or ask for an Extension to file.

On the other hand, some important tasks (such as elective surgery or saving for retirement) are put on the 'backburner' for as long as possible. Note that many people may consider these as unpleasant chores involving 'up-front' financial outlays and/or psychic pain.

Consequently, procrastination seems like a way out.

Here is their rationale:

Why should I do unpleasant tasks now if I can avoid or put them off?

Thus, procrastination typically involves delaying unpleasant decisions/actions until they become truly urgent. The essential aspect of procrastinating is to postpone consideration of an issue until it cannot wait any longer. It has one or more of the following characteristics:

1. Delay action for the time being.
2. Postpone any serious consideration for a more opportune time.
3. Hope that the problem will go away sooner or later.
4. If the task is unpleasant, don't bother doing it now.
5. Lack of interest in carrying out a necessary chore as in "I don't feel like doing it right now; it can wait."

Discussion:

Procrastination can be an entrenched habit or a personal trait regardless of the nature of the task. It amounts to completely turning around the age-old maxim 'Do not wait until tomorrow what should be done today' into "If you can do it later, why bother to do it now?"

There are many essential tasks (albeit unpleasant or boring) as well as unavoidable obligations which we all need to attend to. Procrastinators find many reasons or excuses to postpone them. They just wait and keep putting off those tasks until the last possible moment.

One must make a clear distinction between procrastination and postponement. The latter strategy is legitimate when (a) you need additional information to make an informed decision (b) the subject under consideration is weighty.

Rationale for Procrastination:
Doing an especially unpleasant task takes away resources from other more desirable activities.

Whenever there is no immediate payoff from doing a chore or very little penalty for not doing it soon, there is a good excuse/tendency to put it off. Some procrastinators get a 'kick' out of waiting and even make a 'virtue' of it—you might almost say they enjoy doing so.

Inertia, laziness, and the natural tendency to occupy oneself with more pleasant and satisfying activities can justify procrastinating. Whenever you are called upon to execute a task which is time-consuming, difficult, boring, or psychologically painful—it becomes a good candidate for procrastination.

This is often a pre-programmed and conditional reflex—automatic, habitual, and unconscious. In other words, procrastination is the de-facto decision.

Or it may be the result of a conscious, deliberate, cost-benefit calculation, a proven strategy based on previous experience. In some cases, this can be a smart, convenient, and justifiable course of action.

Sometimes procrastinators stand ready and willing to bear the costs of delayed action. They may also benefit from such strategic waiting as when a 'last-minute bargain' turns up or the necessity for appropriate action no longer exists.

Here are some examples at justification—whether or not they are convincing:

i. I can't afford the expense right now; maybe prices will come down after the holidays.

ii. We don't have enough time to do the job during this holiday season. We will take it up next year.

iii. This project can wait for a while; it is time-consuming; there is no big advantage in rushing to complete it right now. I will get to it when I have more time.

iv. Perhaps this health/medical problem will go away by itself; if not, there is still plenty of time to take care of it.

Concluding Comments:

Habitual procrastinators who desire to change their ways can look back and try to evaluate how much they gained or lost from procrastinating. When you confront similar situations in the future(as often happens), a sincere effort can be made to change your behavior.

For example, you can reward yourself for not procrastinating in different ways. Reward yourself generously and repeatedly. The reward system can be financial, psychological or something very meaningful to you. The very prospect of relief from stress should be uplifting! The joy that comes from a job well done and approbation from those you love and respect can boost your spirits. Such a self-imposed behavior modification strategy can work wonders for your psychic wellbeing. Reinforced by repeated successes (keeping the 'demon of procrastination' at bay), you will be able to get rid of this entrenched habit.

Negative incentives can also work. Punishing yourself—with sincerity—for future lapses can help when the 'punishment is right.' For example, you can give up something you really enjoy (that second cup of morning coffee)—or contribute to a charity you dislike. The prospect of having to do such unpleasant things can probably serve as a 'wake-up call,' which is really what you want.

Select whichever 'negative incentive' works for you—this is a personal choice. You can subject yourself to any suitable system of rewards and punishments with the object of freeing yourself from habitual procrastination—a worthy goal indeed.

Window Dressing or the Art of Selective Information Disclosure:

Whenever someone presents critical information or articles for sale in a positive, pleasing format to influence your opinion/decision, it is a case of 'window dressing.' In such situations, there may be calculated elements of exaggeration about the merits of a product/service—at times, even deliberate distortion of facts or withholding of certain information which may be considered unfavorable.

This is a classic form of presentation designed to impress the customer. Readers may be familiar with seeing pictures of well-dressed, beautifully decorated mannequins on shop windows during the Christmas holiday season. Such colorful, attractive displays convey many desirable attributes of a product to make a favorable impression. Extensive use of such 'window dressing' techniques are employed by advertisers to influence consumer purchasing decisions.

Such presentations sometimes constitute what economists call 'asymmetric information.' In this situation, one party to a transaction (usually the seller) has more information about the underlying product than the other party (a potential buyer). Relevant, vital information (considered unfavorable) is selectively withheld (or not revealed) to make a quick sale. Examples abound:

When one party to a transaction possesses more pertinent information about the item being transacted than the other—as usually happens with the owner/seller of a house/car—vis-à-vis the potential buyer, we have a case of asymmetric information.

This may put the buyer at a disadvantage, especially when information relevant to the transaction is not revealed to the buyer.

1. Some stockbrokers (especially "cold callers") provide only selective information about the past performance of a certain stock or mutual fund. Statistics are presented in such a way as to highlight the positive, favorable aspects of the underlying security and any unfavorable information lies hidden in the background—often referred to as 'the fine print,' which is difficult to comprehend.

2. In romantic encounters, especially on a 'first date,' each party attempts to present themselves to the other as especially desirable or attractive, revealing only their positive, most desirable attributes.

3. Car dealers typically use language such as "Excellent gas mileage, low maintenance costs, 0% interest-rate financing, instant cash rebates" to promote sales of otherwise slow-moving models which typically have limited consumer interest.

4. Such 'underestimation of costs' constitutes an example of asymmetric information because the buyer may be unable to verify the relevant data.

In these cases, the maxim "Let the Buyer Beware" is especially pertinent.

I used to wonder why some people I know, who have a lot of good things going for them—among these I count good health, a well-paying job, financial wherewithal and a decent family life—feel unhappy and dissatisfied with their lot. At the same time, some folks who have little in the way of material wellbeing or emotional support seemed to be content with their lot in life. This is an interesting and perplexing phenomenon. Here are the main differences between these two groups:

Table 5: Some Personal Traits & Behavioral Patterns

Positive/Favorable	Negative/Unfavorable
Consider their glasses 'half-full'	Glasses are half-empty
Count their blessings	Bemoan their misfortune
Light a candle to remove the darkness	Curse the prevailing darkness
Work hard to get what they want	Complain how bad things are
Make do with what they have	There is never enough
Take 'proactive' steps to avoid breakdown/mishaps	Wait until breakdowns occur
Prepare for the uncertain future	Put off action until later
Do regular exercise/eat nutritious food	Often lead unhealthy lives
Save regularly & automatically	Nothing left to save after expenses
Offer help & support to those in need	Think mostly about their own needs
Exercise self-control/discipline	Shift blame elsewhere

Note: This is a simple-minded attempt to explain how people's attitudes often shape their views and influence decision/actions. It is not meant to be a full explanation of what makes 'people tick'.

Ignorance is one of the root causes of poor decisions.

Imagine if you are trying to find a lost key in the dark: it is going to be very hard and probably doomed to fail.

If you are driving without a road map (nowadays without a GPS), you are likely to get lost before reaching your destination. You will be wasting a lot of resources—time, gasoline (money) and mental energy.

If you are going to fight a war, you need the right weapons. And careful planning as well as an appropriate strategy to defeat the enemy; otherwise, the chances of winning could be abysmally low.

Making a decision without sufficient and relevant information is akin to these examples. Good decision-making, under the best of circumstances, is a challenging task. The success of a decision depends on how well-informed you are about its pros and cons or benefits and costs. Ideally, decision-makers should aim to achieve their expected objectives with a minimum expenditure of resources.

When you must make financial decisions without sufficient 'financial know-how,' you are at a tremendous disadvantage. You will end up incurring higher costs and getting lower returns.

Many research studies have shown that people who make financial decisions—buying, selling, borrowing, lending, saving, investing, and conducting transactions in the mortgage markets—end up paying a heavy price for their 'financial illiteracy.' In a nutshell, they put themselves at a great disadvantage. They end up paying higher prices when they buy and get lower prices when they sell. They get subpar returns on investments and pay higher interest rates on mortgages. They also incur higher costs when they seek financial services of all kinds—banking, insurance, investment products and management fees.

There are many reasons for this state of affairs. Here are a few:

1. Lack of familiarity with financial markets and how they function.
2. Ignorance of transaction costs and their impact on investment returns.
3. Not understanding the significance of how small changes in the term structure of interest rates profoundly influence mortgage costs.

Financial Decisions

An important area of decision-making concerns lifetime money management. Whether you are young or old, employed or unemployed, single or head of a family, wealthy or poor, working or retired, everyone needs to manage their financial resources as efficiently as possible. This requires a certain amount of financial literacy and familiarity with financial markets in general.

A brief introduction to financial markets is provided here.

A considerable amount of money will be flowing through your hands during the lifecycle. Here is a rough breakdown of what this looked like in 2020.

Table 6: Education & Income

Education Level	Lifetime Income
Less than high school education:	1.2-2.2 million
High school	1.9-2.4
Some college	1.8-2.7
Bachelor's degree	2.7-3.7
Graduate degree	3.4-4.2
Professional degree	4.2-5.4

These estimates are based on average annual incomes for each educational cohort multiplied by (roughly) 40-50 years of working life (Source: Federal Reserve; Social Security Adm., 2020).

Undoubtedly, being able to manage this cashflow diligently will greatly enhance your financial wellbeing. Regardless of how much or how little money you earn or inherit during your lifetime, people without some financial savvy will be hard put to meet this challenge. One must therefore become familiar with certain rudimentary principles of finance. Unfortunately, even many college graduates are woefully lacking in this respect. We will now familiarize readers with some basic financial vocabulary.

A. Stocks and Flows

The term 'Stock' means any quantity of something that already exists at a moment in time, such as your bank balance on January 1, 2021, or the value of your investment portfolio on December 31, 2021. This 'stock' signifies a fixed quantity, akin to the number of books in a library or a photograph of yourself on your 20th birthday. The word 'Flow,' on the other hand, is like a movie with changing scenes from moment to moment. Or the flow of water in a river on a given day.

Your salary or income is a periodic payment (flow), measured per unit of time such as a week, month, or year. When you save a portion of your monthly income for future use, it is added to the stock of wealth you have already saved. This is one of the ways in which wealth accumulates over a period of time—the other factor being the effect of compound interest.

Note that some portion of the flow of periodic income is turned into a stock of wealth with the act of saving. When decisions are made to defer or postpone spending of current income, a transfer of purchasing power takes place from now to the future. This is how wealth can be built up over your lifetime.

B. Income and Wealth

Income refers to a constant, continuous, or periodic flow of money measured over a specific time interval—such as a week, month, or year. Most workers are paid a wage or salary weekly or monthly, in the form of a paycheck (cash flow). If you own rental property, you earn 'rent,' which constitutes a periodic flow of income. Likewise, 'dividends' represent periodic (Quarterly) payments of income to stockholders. 'Interest income' is earned by those who have loaned money to others for a certain period of time. Bondholders or those who own savings accounts collect such periodic interest payments from debtors such as banks, corporations or government entities.

These periodic income flows enable millions of recipients to spend or save. When you decide to save a certain portion of this cash flow, it adds to your stock of wealth, making it available for potential future use. Any periodic income flow can be spent now or saved for the future, depending on what you decide to do with it. This is an important allocation decision which eventually determines your overall lifetime income stream—with many ramifications.

C. Human Capital

An individual's potential lifetime earning power depends on the quantity and quality of education, skills and know-how embodied in that person. (Embodied means integral or inseparable.) People who have acquired specialized practical knowledge and problem-solving skills of all kinds—represented by their educational attainments, practical training, and work experience—will command high levels of income in a competitive labor market. Thus Human Capital can add significantly to one's earning power as it is highly valued by employers. (Some economists compare these 'earnings' to a 'bond-like' income stream with the only difference that while bonds can be bought and sold in the financial markets, endowed 'human capital' is nontransferable.)

The amount of income passing through your hands during a lifetime of work—roughly 40 to 50 years—depends on when you decide to join the labor force and when you decide to quit working. As stated earlier, this income stream can range between a minimum of 1.50 million ($30,000 x 50 years) for a high school graduate, and upwards of $5 million ($125,000 x 40 years) for a professional degree holder. These figures are probably underestimates in today's technologically sophisticated and rapidly growing economic environment where human capital is a highly prized asset.

It is incumbent on you to manage this enormous flow of income stream by making smart, judicious spending and saving decisions. This means among other things: (a) knowing not only how to earn, but more importantly, (b) how to spend, save, borrow, lend, invest, accumulate, and manage that money. Inability or failure to do so can result in unnecessary and avoidable financial distress. To help readers on this somewhat tricky and challenging road called 'lifetime money management,' here are some helpful hints and suggestions.

1. Allocation of Current Income between Spending and Saving:
Regardless of how low or high one's income level happens to be, most people have a hard time finding enough (spare) cash to put away for their future needs. It is ironic that some families making $200,000-$300,000 per month in some wealthy American cities and suburbs—roughly the top 10% of the U.S. income pyramid!—cannot balance their budgets. They too 'complain' about their financial struggles and challenges. There is a constant tug-of-war going on in their lives between the very pressing needs (wants?) of the present vis-à-vis providing for an uncertain, distant future. It is important to strike a judicious balance between your well-deserved and worthy aspirations to enjoy a decent lifestyle now, while still making some prudent allowance for a leisurely but uncertain 'retirement lifespan'—waiting in the wings.

Between these two polar opposites, there could be some other pressing needs, requiring you to allocate current income for:

(a) An 'emergency fund' for unplanned and
    unexpected expenses: 3%

(b) Annual or periodic vacations/travel   2%

(c) Repairs, or planned replacements of home   3%
    appliances/automobiles, furniture, etc.

(d) Education (college savings fund)   2%

(e) Prospective retirement contributions   10%

Total Savings:

                                                20% of
                                                current income

As you can see, by adding up these five categories (based on household expenditure surveys), one might plan for a target saving rate of about 20%. (Some financial experts label this strategy as the 50/30/20 rule of spending, meaning: 50% for basic items such as food, clothing, and household expenses; 30% for discretionary items and 20% for saving.) In fact, for those individuals/families with seasonally fluctuating incomes, the 'cash cushion' needs to be even greater. Adhering to this prudent saving strategy will ensure your being able to ride out temporary layoffs, unexpected large medical bills, or other financial setbacks—which happen to occur at the most inconvenient time. Setting up an appropriate saving arrangement with your bank/financial institution, working automatically and seamlessly, will be a smart, proactive decision.

D. Assets, Liabilities & Net Worth:

Periodic assessment of where you stand financially is akin to our annual physical checkups—they can provide important clues about your overall financial health and wellbeing. Smart money management involves reviewing your financial position at least once every year. This can be done in two steps. First, list all your 'assets'—such as real estate, bank accounts, savings, stock and bond holdings, IRAs, retirement accounts, etc. Second, make a complete list of all your 'liabilities'—financial obligation such as: home mortgages, car loans, credit card balances, personal/equipment/travel loans, unpaid bills/taxes, and money owed to others.

Now you are ready to compute your 'net worth' at the end of the year. Assets – Liabilities = Net Worth

This number is an index of your overall financial health. It should be reviewed annually (or more often) to make sure that you are making satisfactory progress toward achieving financial independence. Reasons for lack of progress, if any, can then be assessed and remedied.

E. Debt Management

Individuals, households, businesses, and various private/governmental bodies often experience significant gaps between current income (cash flow or receipts) and current expenditures or payments. Since periodic receipts and payments seldom match, there results either a Surplus (excess of income over current expenditures) or Deficit (expenses exceed income).

We can designate financial entities as either surplus or deficit units, depending on their periodic cash flow status. Surplus units have no use for their current savings. They are ready and willing to part with this surplus at least temporarily. Deficit units are looking for funds to bridge the gap between current payments and receipts.

Notice that the same economic entity, say your household, can be a surplus unit at one time and a deficit unit later on. For example, if you are short of funds to buy a car, you need to borrow money to come up with the initial 'down-payment' as well as monthly instalment payments. Likewise, when you are saving a portion of your current income for future needs, you are willing and able to lend this surplus to others—through the intermediation of financial markets.

This is where the 'Market for Debt Instruments' enters the picture.

Savers are seeking an outlet to lend their surplus funds to borrowers to earn interest income—a compensation or reward for parting with their 'current liquidity.' Explanation: Money or cash has the quality of being extremely liquid—or has liquidity—a term used by economists to signify its ready, universal acceptability for all financial transactions. When you lend money, you are temporarily converting this liquidity into 'illiquidity' and signaling your willingness to postpone current spending. This enables a potential borrower to use those funds to finance their temporary deficits. The longer the period for which you are willing to lend (postpone your own spending), the greater the degree of illiquidity. The prevailing interest rates for different durations of loans—reflect the scarcity or abundance of liquidity. Thus, while lenders (surplus units) seek compensation for parting with their liquidity, borrowers are willing to pay interest for the privilege of using that money. The length/term of the loan period determines the appropriate interest rate, which is based on the availability (supply) of loanable funds in relation to the demand for those funds at any given time.

Like any other market-determined price, the interaction of supply and demand for loanable funds determines the prevailing interest rates. Those rates can frequently go up or down, to bring about balance between savings and borrowings.

There are many other factors which influence the interest rates you pay or receive as a consumer/household/saver/lender. They include:

(a) Where and with whom you are conducting your business/transaction. Financial markets can be segmented locally or nationally. Are you dealing with a local bank/credit union, or do you have access to a wider network of financial institutions operating nationally or internationally?

(b) Risk parameters of the transaction—your creditworthiness as reflected in your FICO score and other relevant factors.

(c) The principal amount as well as the term-period of the loan.

(d) Whether the interest rate is fixed or floating (tied to an index).

Note that the market for financial instruments is large, complex, volatile, widespread, and extremely fluid. You have plenty of choices and opportunities to make use of them to suit your specific needs and interests. In general, most consumers/households act as Price-takers, meaning that they must accept and settle for the prevailing market conditions/interest rates and loan parameters whether you are a lender or borrower.

F. Risk and Reward

It is one of the axioms of finance that 'risk and reward' are inversely related. This means that the higher the riskiness of an investment, the greater is the expected reward. This principle is illustrated in the following diagram:

Figure 10:

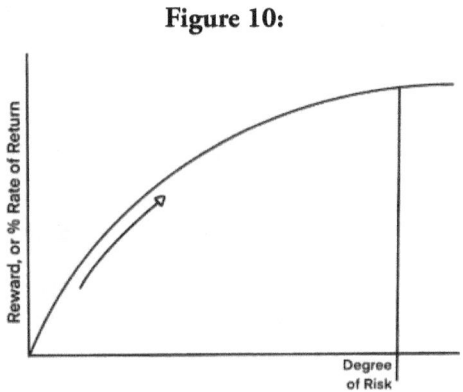

Notice that the risk/reward ratio rises rapidly at first and flattens out as you move along the risk spectrum. Beyond a certain point, taking greater risk does not automatically increase reward. As a general rule, those seeking a higher reward must be willing to take greater risk—with the probability that you may not fully recover the capital invested.

Types of Debt Instruments:
Well-established business organizations and governmental bodies can usually borrow money by issuing debt instruments called Bonds. These bonds represent promises to pay back the money borrowed at some future date. The borrowing entities promise to pay a certain rate of interest

on such bonds. The interest rate depends on their credit worthiness—
which reflects their marketability. There is a well-established market for
all types of bonds issued by corporations as well as government agencies.
Bond-rating agencies such as Moodys or Standard & Poor determine the
creditworthiness of different borrowers, based on various criteria. Therefore, a typical bond buyer can be reasonably certain that the 'coupon
rate' of a bond reflects its overall credit quality. In general, bonds carrying
AAA (top-rated) rating represent the top of the bond pyramid. Bonds
with lower rating carry higher interest rates to compensate for their extra
risk. This tier arrangement allows lenders (bond buyers) to pick and
choose what type of bonds are appropriate for their portfolios.

The market for debt instruments of various types is huge. The U.S.
Government is the largest borrower in the world. The 30-year U.S. Government bond is used as a benchmark for measuring prevailing credit
conditions for all other long-term bonds.

Retail buyers such as households can buy and sell most bonds
through a broker. U.S. Government securities can sometimes be purchased through a bank. It is also possible to set up a direct purchase account with the Treasury if you plan to hold them for long periods.

G. Compound Interest

Albert Einstein is reputed to have said: "Compound interest is the 8th
wonder of the world." Here is why.

When you borrow money, you pay interest on the loan. Likewise,
when you save and invest, you receive interest. The interest you pay or receive is called 'simple interest.' It is calculated as a percentage of the 'principal' per unit of time—usually per year. For example, $100 borrowed for

one year at 6% simple interest earns $6. If the loan is extended for another year, the interest cost becomes $12. At the end of a twelve-year period, the borrower must repay $172: the principal of $100 + accumulated interest of $72 ($6% per year x 12 years = $72).

With Compound Interest, the method of calculating interest is different. The interest rate is 'compounded every year,' meaning that the interest earned in the first year also earns interest in the second and subsequent years. Thus, the twelve-year loan at 6% compound interest will end up earning a total of almost $100 in accumulated interest— rather than only $72 as in the case of simple interest. Notice that the difference between $100 – 72 = 28 is the result of earning 'interest on interest'— the effect of compounding.

Figure 11: Growth Rates and Accumulated Savings

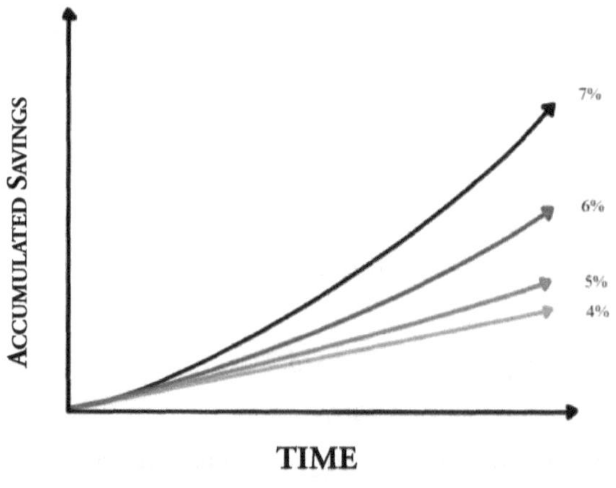

The higher the interest rate and the greater the number of periods of compounding, the greater becomes the difference between simple and compound interest rates. This 'magic' effect of compounding can best be understood with the so-called "Rule of 72."

According to this rule, the number of years needed for any entity to double in value can be calculated by:

$$72/i = n$$

Where i = the rate of interest or growth rate
n = number of years of compounding

Thus, in the previous example of 6% compound interest and a 12 year loan, the original $100 doubles in value to $200.

Here is a table illustrating how an investment of $100 doubles in value. Notice that the higher the growth rate, the lesser is the time needed for the principal to double.

Table 7: Impact of Different Growth Rates on Income

Growth Rate	Number of Years	Final Value
4%	18	200
6%	12	200
8%	9	200
10%	7.2	200
12%	6	200

Example: If you invest $1000 at age 20, growing at 6% compounded, you will have $16,000 at age 68.

If you can generate an 8% growth rate on the same initial investment, you can harvest $32,000! As you can see, compound interest can produce astronomical growth over long periods of time.

High growth rates, combined with longer time periods, can create enormous amounts of wealth. This is why money management/retirement planning outfits such as Vanguard, Fidelity and T. Rowe Price encourage young workers and investors to start saving for their retirement as early as possible. The following example demonstrates the superiority of this simple investment strategy.

Figure 12

How Starting to Invest Early Pays Handsomely

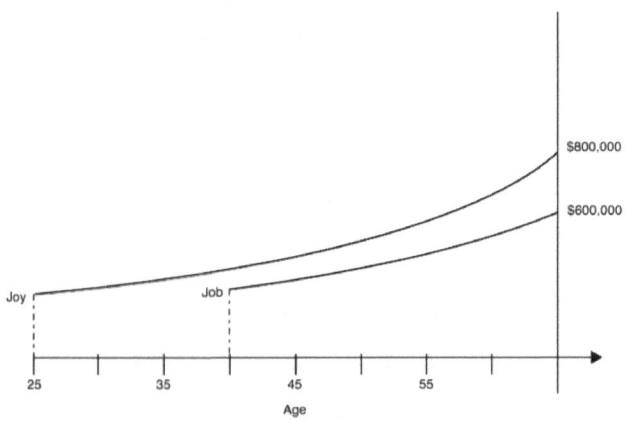

Source: This Diagram is based on a similar presentation by TIAA.
Joy invests $5,000 annually, stating at age 25
Job invests $10,000 annually, stating at age 40
At age 65, Joy has accumulated $200,000 more than Job

Notice that although Job has invested $50,000 more than Joy overall, he ends up with $200,000 LESS at age 65. This difference is attributable to: (1) Joy having started to invest at an earlier age, (2) which provided her significantly more time to reap the benefits of compounding.

H. Risk and Safety

Many a time, decisions must be made under the cloak of uncertainty. In addition to the many challenges of making decisions when all pertinent facts and information are readily available, uncertainty throws an additional wrench into the equation.

When the probability of an adverse event can be reasonably quantified, one can buy insurance for protection against losses. This is an aspect of Risk Management. With the right kind of insurance, an insurer guarantees that you will be protected against events such as: damage to property, ill health, disability, unemployment, and other types of hazards that can result in financial losses. What types of risks you want to insure against and how much premium you are willing to pay to offset those risks, depend on your personal circumstances.

When the outcome of an event is unknown and unpredictable, it is referred to as 'uncertainty.' Since uncertainty cannot be easily quantified, one must be prepared to bear the associated risks, in cases such as:

(a) A surgery where the doctor warns you against potential failure/ complications but expects a reasonable degree of success.
(b) A promising, new experimental medical treatment which may not work as expected or can cause unspecified adverse results.

c) The price of a stock may go up or down after your purchase—there is uncertainty about the direction it will take.

(d) You may pass or fail a driving test; win or lose a game.

(e) Your opponent in the witness stand may be telling the truth or lying (we do not know which).

In all such cases, it is up to you, the decision-maker, to shoulder the risks associated with possible adverse outcomes. Here are some strategies for consideration.

I. Risk Tolerance

How much risk can you tolerate? What is your attitude to risk?

People's attitude to risk varies over a wide spectrum depending on their personality types. Here are some common categories.

a. Extreme Risk Aversion

Those who perceive certain situations as especially risky tend to avoid them by choosing not to participate in those activities. Common examples are fear of flying or fear of heights (some choose to call this a phobia).

The risk of losing money—even a small fraction of their invested capital, can keep some folks away from the stock market. According to what is known as 'Prospect Theory,' the loss of a dollar is generally twice as painful as the pleasure derived from gaining a dollar.

Extreme risk aversion (seeking safety at any cost) can be detrimental to one's financial wellbeing. It can also limit your freedom of action in many fields of endeavor, denying oneself pleasurable and profitable opportunities which are available to others.

b.   Moderate Risk Aversion

Some degree of risk is inherent in almost everything we do. It is a fact of life. There is really no escape from this reality. The question is: How much risk are you willing to shoulder?

Most people address this question in a practical way. This is because buying protective insurance can be expensive, beyond some level of risk. They choose to buy insurance against catastrophic losses and 'self-insure' against moderate or small losses which they can afford to bear.

c. Risk Lovers are those who seek and embrace risky situations which others shun or consider unacceptable. They enjoy the thrill, challenge and adventure associated with taking on risky undertakings. They know that risky investments, on average, produce higher financial rewards and are willing to bet on them.

Those who are willing to bear higher than normal risks in their job environment—miners, divers, workers dealing with hazardous/toxic materials or explosives, window-washers of high-rise buildings, etc., are rewarded by higher wages proportionate to the degree of risk.

Extreme risk taking is common among certain sports enthusiasts and lovers of recreational activities. Skydiving, bungee jumping, high-wire acts, speed car racing, remote mountaineering and performing certain stunts are examples of such behavior.

J. The Measurement of Risk

There are different parameters for measuring risk. The commonly used statistical term is known as standard deviation (SD). It is a measure of how far an individual's position lies above or below the mean of a normal distribution. For example, suppose the mean SAT score among female college applicants is 1,500, with a standard deviation of 150. If Emily's score is 1,800, she is two SDs above the mean. The probability of having a score as high as 1,800 is less than 2.5%.

Figure 13

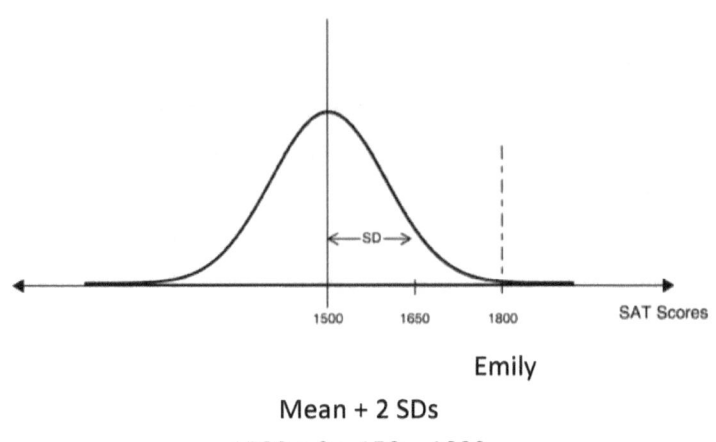

The Normal Distribution (or Bell Curve)

1500   1650   1800   SAT Scores

Emily

Mean + 2 SDs

1500 + 2 x 150 = 1800

In other words, 95% of all SAT scores will lie within a range of 1,200 to 1,800—i.e.: within 1.96 SDs from the mean for that normal distribution. (Some 'selective colleges' may admit only applicants in the top 5% of the SAT distribution.)

Similarly, readers may be familiar with a widely used measure of a person's credit rating, known as the FICO score. Suppose the mean FICO score is 630 with a SD of 70. When you apply for a mortgage, one of the criteria used by potential lenders is your creditworthiness. If your FICO score happens to be 745, you are just a hair breadth above 1.65 SDs above the average. This means you belong to the top 5% of all loan applicants. Many lenders use some predetermined 'cut off' FICO scores to determine your eligibility for the best mortgage rates.

Note: The FICO score does not follow a normal distribution.

Another interpretation of risk is the degree of volatility—ups and downs—commonly found in the fluctuating price of a financial asset. Highly volatile stocks tend to have a high 'beta' score. Those who generally seek safety stick to investing in 'low beta' financial instruments (with AAA or similar ratings). Investors who seek above average rewards accept the risks associated with highly volatile stocks or lower-quality bonds with ratings below B or B-.

K. Controlling, Minimizing and Managing Risk

Risks can be managed in different ways. The main idea here is to 'manage'—not eliminate.

The techniques used to manage risk depend on the magnitude and character of the underlying risk. The two common methods are:

(a) Pooling of Risk through Diversification.

This approach to risk management is commonly employed when you want protection against wild price fluctuations in a single asset class. By investing in different types of assets (with differing risk characteristics), one can minimize overall portfolio risk. For example, if you are saving for retirement, you could use different proportions of:

- Domestic and foreign stocks, large and small
- Government and corporate bonds, long- and short-term
- Real estate investment trusts—office, commercial, residential
- Precious metals and commodities
- Money market instruments, etc.

NOTE: Your current age, appetite for risk, and time horizon should determine the combinations and characteristics of these assets—known as 'Asset Allocation Decision' strategy.

(b) Purchasing insurance is the most common risk management strategy used by households/businesses. Buying insurance shifts various types of risks from the buyer to the insurance underwriter.

Whether and how much insurance protection to buy is a decision you must ponder carefully. Here are some basic guidelines:

1. What is the nature and magnitude of the specific risk? Is it catastrophic? such as damage to life and property.
2. How much of this potential risk should or can you afford to shoulder—called 'self-insurance'?
3. What is the premium cost in relation to the potential monetary benefit if you make a 'claim'? Is the premium reasonable and affordable?
4. Are you required by law to purchase this insurance? (e.g., automobile liability)
5. How much 'insurable interest' (ownership) do you have in this asset?
6. What would happen if you did not buy insurance protection? You are then 'self-insuring' the entire risk.

Discussion:

Catastrophic means those (huge, almost unbearable) losses which would materially impair your financial wellbeing. If you are strongly 'risk averse,' you should buy enough insurance to protect your financial interests.

To keep the premium costs low, you can opt for as high a 'deductible' as you can live with. The higher this 'self-insurance' element, the lower the premium will be. The premium cost, as a percentage of insurance coverage, should be kept low (a benchmark)—around 5% or less.

Certain types of insurance may be mandated by law. Examples are:

a) Flood insurance (for homes located in a flood-designated area).
b) Automobile liability & property damage.
c) Lien-holder policy mandated by a lender.
d) Secondary mortgage insurance—required by lenders when the total mortgage amount exceeds 80% of the property value.
e) Health insurance—a necessity: The type of coverage available to you and its 'affordability' vary widely, depending on age and your state of health.
f) Insurable interest refers to anyone who may have exposure to financial risks, with a stake in the underlying asset.

As a rule of thumb, certain types of insurance are best avoided, provided you are willing and able to bear the associated risks. This is because the premium costs can be prohibitively high in relation to the risks covered. Such insurance is sometimes aggressively marketed and promoted—you guessed it—on 'naïve,' unsuspecting beneficiaries and the elderly.

These policies only cover minimal or almost 'non'-existent' risks, designed to make money for sellers of insurance: not the buyers.

Here are the classic examples:

i. Flight insurance: The risk of dying in a plane crash is infinitesimally low.
ii. Credit card insurance: This is unnecessary—you are only liable for a maximum of $50 for fraudulent use of your card by others.
iii. Life insurance on young children: They are not wage-earners. You don't depend on them for your livelihood— although they are priceless emotionally.
iv. Certain 'high-cost' travel insurance plans: Buy them very carefully and examine the 'fine print' before doing so. The premium cost can be a high percentage of the insurance's face value and the probability of 'collecting' is low.

Relationship between Risk & Reward

The typical individual is risk averse. Normally everyone would prefer safety over risk if the rewards were identical. Therefore, those who take on more risk can normally expect to be rewarded for doing so. This 'risk premium' depends on many factors: in general, the higher the degree of risk, the higher is the associated reward. Without such additional compensation, no one will assume greater risk.

Here are some guidelines:

(1) As mentioned earlier, workers engaged in occupations considered as risky (handling hazardous materials) will command higher wage rates than workers in relatively 'safe' jobs.

(2) Corporate bonds sold by less creditworthy firms (also called 'junk bonds') carry higher interest rates than those with higher credit rating (AAA).

(3) Long-term bonds, which are exposed to higher 'interest rate risk'—because of their longevity—command higher interest rates than short-term bonds with similar characteristics.

Conclusion: Those who are searching for higher yields/rates of return must be prepared to accept commensurately above average risks. This is an inevitable trade-off. It is up to you to choose the appropriate risk/reward ratio that provides the peace of mind and financial wellbeing that you seek.

The High Cost of Safety

Though insurance provides protection against different hazards and risks, one should guard against seeking 'excessive safety.' Trying to protect yourself against every conceivable risk can be prohibitively expensive. One should be judicious in buying insurance because premiums can add up fast, taking a toll on your budget. Let me give some examples:

1. As you age, and life expectancy decreases, life insurance premiums increase disproportionately.
2. Automobile premiums for collision and comprehensive coverage become uneconomical for older cars.
3. It is generally advisable and economical to opt for a 'larger deductible'—at least $1,000—on property insurance (houses/

cars). The reason is that cumulative annual savings in premiums would more than compensate for an occasional 'out-of-pocket' expense. (Ask yourself: how many insurance claims have you made in the last ten years for property damage?)

4. As a 'rule of thumb,' one should seek out the lowest premium cost in relation to the risks covered. Insurance is designed to protect against large, catastrophic losses. Making frequent claims for small damages will end up costing more in premium payments and will soon become uneconomical.

A Digression on Advisors, Life Coaches, Counsellors, Guides, Gurus, and Sages

As we have seen, one of the remarkable features of modern life is the availability of outsourcing opportunities to carry out various tasks that you are unable or unwilling to do yourself. If you can pay someone to do what you don't want to do, they will be more than willing to oblige for the right price.

In this internet age, a plethora of outsourcing businesses have sprung up throughout the land to cater to burgeoning demand. You can find experts eager to help with whatever problem you entrust to them, at a price. This includes help and advice on making decisions about any conceivable subject—education, career choice, marital problems, financial planning, healthy lifestyles, retirement issues, sex, personal relationships, recreational activities, travel—ad nfinitum.

You will have to determine how useful, practical, reliable, and valuable such advice is: and how much and for how long you can afford to pay for these advisory services.

When you want to deal with ongoing, complex issues such as prolonged health problems, legal affairs or resolve end-of-life legacy matters—it is certainly advisable to seek expert guidance.

How do you define or measure success?

A successful life is what everyone wants and hopes for.

There are many possible interpretations of 'success.' It has multiple dimensions: some visible and measurable; others hidden, but very meaningful.

Success is often associated with desirable outcomes—such as securing material wealth, fame, fortune, awards, credentials, promotions, winning elections or competitive games, love, and satisfaction with your accomplishments in life.

Another dimension of success is: Being able to serve society and devote oneself to solving social/environmental problems. Great personal and emotional satisfaction can spring from helping others in need—sharing and caring — especially in professions such as education/ medicine/ healthcare/ social welfare/ counseling/public health advocacy/ and many nonprofit sectors. People who follow their 'passion' to serve society—regardless of financial rewards—belong to this category.

Being able to do what you want, when you want, where you want, on your terms, is the paramount goal of 'free-to-be' individuals. To them, success is measured by the degree of freedom they enjoy, pursuing their personal interests—climbing mountains, exploring wilderness areas, rescuing distressed/endangered animals, walking, cycling, or sailing around the world—being engaged in doing what they consider rewarding and fulfilling.

There is another aspect of success which is worth exploring. It is often invisible and defies measurement. For some individuals, the mere act of survival and striving to overcome everyday obstacles is a herculean task. For example, getting out of poverty and becoming financially self- sufficient is a true measure of success for children born in poor households. If one is afraid of heights, being able to climb a ladder, tree, or other tall structures can be considered as success. Overcoming the many hurdles, obstacles, and challenges that you confront on the road to a fulfilling life, is the hallmark of success. For those who are disabled and find it difficult to walk, talk, hear, see, or move their limbs, being able to perform many ordinary tasks by exercising their willpower is success indeed.

Success can mean winning an argument or persuading a reluctant spouse (or opponent) to agree with your point of view. It is the ability to convince others that you can transcend difficulties that stand in the way of completing a certain task or assignment. When failure stares you in the face, summoning enough courage and marshalling the necessary resources to get the job done is the hallmark of success.

Not succumbing to discouragement, loss, failure, unjust criticism, or other hurdles but focusing on reaching the ultimate goal, contributes to success.

Believing in oneself, and not giving up when 'the going gets tough,' requires courage, patience, and endurance. These are qualities that lead to success in any endeavor. Self-respect, self-confidence, self-control, and self-reliance are the pillars on which successful people rely to build their lives.

Even if you have tried and failed many times, but still convinced that you can reach your goal in the next attempt, you embody the true spirit of success. It is ultimately a mental attitude, a mindset, a formidable hidden power which accompanies you wherever you choose to go.

Success means you go about pursuing your goals and dreams whether there is light or darkness. You take calculated risks. You work hard with earnest discipline and commitment. You motivate yourself to get what you want to achieve. You do not surrender or give up. You succeed regardless of any obstacles put in front of you. And try to get what you want. Your temperament, attitude and outlook must be geared to achieve what you set out to do. When others criticize or discourage you, ignore them. Show them what you can do.

Measure progress daily. Take small steps. Be glad if you are making steady progress. Reward yourself for small accomplishments. Pat yourself. Stay calm when disappointments happen and smile. Go about your tasks leisurely. Don't rush. There is no hurry. Take your time and enjoy what you are doing.

Success means you live your life on your own terms. You are not beholden to any particular dogma. You set your own rules and play the game accordingly. You push the ball slowly, steadily, bit by bit until it reaches where you want it to go.

You stay focused. Even if there is no visible progress, you continue to work relentlessly. That is all there is to it.

Your abilities must be put to the test and only you can do it. You know your limitations; what is achievable and what is beyond your power to achieve. It is your life, your work, your passion, your own striving.

Do what you want. Go for it. Pursue it. Keep going. That is success!

Chapter VII
Summary & Conclusions

The Decision-making Landscape
A Simple Question-Answer Format

I thought it would be useful to present the basic ideas about decision-making in a simple, easy-to-read format, especially for the benefit of young readers who are embarking on this fascinating journey of life. I have tried to keep the dialogue straightforward as well as succinct.

Every one of these questions has been treated at length elsewhere in this book. This format should whet the appetite of readers who are looking for quick answers. Hopefully this should spark their curiosity and desire to explore each topic in greater depth later, at a more leisurely pace.

1. **What is a decision?**
    A decision is a concrete plan of action designed to accomplish a specific task and to reach a predetermined goal.

2. **Why should I make decisions?**
    From birth to death, the journey of life is full of choices and opportunities. How you want to live and what you want to do with your life depend on your decisions. If you don't want to be like a

leaf-in-the-wind, being blown around wherever the wind takes you, you must learn to make up your mind. This is the essence of choosing and deciding.

3. How do you decide?

When presented with many choices, you must know which particular choice meets your needs, based on your tastes, preferences and 'values.' You must think about the benefits and costs of each potential choice and pick the one which best satisfies you.

4. What happens if you can't decide?

You can put off the decision for a later time if the decision is not urgent. Or you can consult someone you trust to help you with the decision. If this is not possible, you can try your best shot at one of the available options, see how it evolves, and learn from this experience.

Learning by doing is a good way to prepare for future decisions.

5. What happens if you are afraid to make any decision and try to avoid the task altogether?

You will continue to wonder what will happen, worry about the problem and, by letting this opportunity to pass, allow chance to determine the outcome.

This outcome may or may not be satisfactory. If it turns out to be both disadvantageous and disagreeable, you might learn a valuable lesson from this episode and be more willing to exercise your judgment next time.

6. What is the best way to arrive at a decision?

Know clearly what the issue is. Know what you want to accomplish. Analyze the problem in terms of how it is going to affect your lifestyle. What are the options available? How do they compare with one another in terms of potential costs and benefits? Is one of them superior to others? If not, which one seems to have a good chance of success? Ponder deeply and make up your mind.

Put sufficient resources behind your decision and implement it with gusto!

7. What are the benefits and costs of making a decision?

Benefits:

You can decide what you want done to solve the problem. You are in the best possible position to judge what matters. You know your mind better than anyone else.

You can take appropriate and cost-effective actions to promote your cherished goals. This is a great opportunity to experiment, which should be welcomed wholeheartedly. You can learn valuable lessons from your decisions, both good and bad, and gain experience for making future choices.

Costs:

Decision-making takes time, effort, energy and resources. Some decisions can be very hard, taxing your mental faculties to the limit. You take responsibility for all the choices you make. If they turn out to be disappointing or produce adverse outcomes, you must be willing to accept them. You cannot 'pass the buck' to somebody else and absolve yourself of responsibility. This is why some people don't want to make important decisions and let 'chance' dictate the outcome.

We live in a society where individuals welcome the opportunity to decide for themselves what they want. Nobody else can do this for you but yourself, so you might as well welcome this opportunity.

8. If I cannot make up my mind, what should I do?

Some tough decisions could be difficult to handle. This is especially true when you are emotionally distressed. There are many situations where you are well-advised to consult an expert: e.g. (1) critical medical decisions, (2) investment choices, (3) pension distributions or Social Security issues, and (4) inheritance/legacy/legal matters. These may require extensive consultations with experts who are knowledgeable in their specialized fields.

Whenever you want to consult experts to decide on an important issue, go ahead. This is a positive step and eminently desirable. Ask people whose judgment you respect. Thereafter, take your time to evaluate their opinions/advice; mull over all the pros and cons and then decide.

9. What happens if I keep on procrastinating?

Even after making a decision, I sometimes fail to follow through with it. I keep wondering what might happen. Probably I am ambivalent about my decision. What should I do to overcome my hesitation to implement the decision?

Unfortunately, this is a common problem. First of all, some folks have a hard time making a definite commitment to any course of action. They hope the problem (issue) will go away or somehow sort itself out. This rarely happens and the situation often gets worse. Then they must deal with the issue under duress, which often results in sub-optimal outcomes.

A decision which is not implemented stays in limbo. This can be a serious problem. The window of opportunity may pass quickly. Future costs can escalate, or the expected benefits could diminish while you wait.

A good example of this is investment decisions. Financial markets move rapidly. Once you have done your homework and made up your mind, don't second guess yourself; take the plunge and move on.

10. What about 'seat of the pants' decisions? Or deciding on a whim? Should every decision undergo a thorough 'cost-benefit analysis' and rigorous thinking?

As a rule, it is best to make sure that you have done the necessary 'homework' before making any major decision, so that you don't blame yourself and later regret any hasty move. But there may be occasions when your gut instinct or initial impressions can be trusted. If the matter under consideration is not 'grave, important, or materially significant,' go ahead and trust your judgment. But be prepared to accept the consequences.

11. Why is it important to get all the relevant facts/information before deciding? What happens if adequate/timely information is unavailable, and I must decide quickly?

This can indeed happen. But insufficient/misleading information can distort your judgment. Even in the best of circumstances, decisions based on all available information can be problematic. Without sufficient, reliable facts at your disposal, it is hard to make a major decision. If you have to 'make do' with situations where you are starved of facts, the best you can do is to hope that you are 'right.' And wait for the results that follow from the decision.

12. What is the essential difference between 'good and bad' decisions?
This depends on how the decision was made. Good decisions are based on adequate information, conducting a careful analysis, weighing all pros and cons, and then making an informed judgment. Decisions made hastily, without proper input, based on hunch and driven by powerful emotions, seldom produce satisfactory results. Also, decisions should not be judged merely by their 'outcomes'; good decisions are based on careful analysis, not 'luck of the draw.'

13. What happens if I don't like my earlier decision? Can I change my mind?
Of course. Decisions are not written in stone. If there is a good reason to modify, alter or abort your earlier decision, go ahead and do it. But make sure the new decision that supplants the earlier one is definitely superior, based on what you know now. This assumes that you have not yet implemented the earlier decision. Also make sure that if the earlier decision involved others, their consent and approval are obtained before altering it.

14. What if I reverse the decision?
Again, it is okay to alter your previous decision. Make sure the reasons for reversing the earlier decision are sound and defensible. Be prepared to justify the new decision.

15. Some folks are genuinely afraid of making any decision. They avoid, postpone, put off, procrastinate and defer to others, rather than commit themselves to a definite course of action. What happens to those who can't or don't want to decide?

These folks are ridden by anxiety, fear or feelings of inadequacy. They take refuge in inaction. They let chance dictate what happens to them. They are currently resigned to this state of affairs. But if they want to, they can learn, just like you and me. It is a matter of slowly building one's self-confidence, learning by doing little by little and gaining experience. Over time, they can become good decision-makers.

16. Is it possible to avoid being tangled in emotions while making certain decisions—such as house buying, college choice, spouse selection or other areas where "emotions" dictate what you like or dislike?

Emotions are certainly a big part of such decisions. Human beings are an amalgam of 'feelings, emotions, likes, dislikes, prejudices and preconceived notions,' while also capable of logical reasoning and good judgment. Therefore, if they choose to, they can change/replace their initial emotional reactions with rational thinking. These two approaches, coming from opposite sides of our brains, can be combined suitably, to arrive at satisfactory decisions. One is not doomed to an 'either or' situation. Wisdom and practicality should tone down purely emotional decisions; otherwise, you may be victimized by your own lack of proper judgment.

In a similar vein:

Do situations such as (1) falling in love with a moody/ temperamental person, (2) initial 'favorable impressions' with a challenging job prospect, (3) a risky (but attractive) investment opportunity or (4) mixed reactions about a newly renovated house up for sale at a bargain price, constitute 'red flags'? Is it best to avoid these situations—giving mixed signals?

There is no 'foolproof' way of assessing such prospects, except to investigate and seek further clarification. The very fact that you are attracted to these 'iffy' prospects indicate that you are adventurous and find them worthy of consideration. So, go ahead, but proceed cautiously and make sure that you are fully satisfied with your potential choices.

17. What happens when you find that you cannot deliver on your promises?

This happens often enough. Situations and circumstances can change. Explain sincerely to the parties affected why the promises you made in good faith cannot be fulfilled. Offer to compensate them in some other way, if at all possible.

18. How important is it to 'win & succeed' in the 'game of life'?

Everyone enjoys winning, succeeding, and getting what you want. Losing, surrendering and accepting failure are painful experiences. However, our decisions and actions must be imbued with good intentions and integrity. They must be ethically and morally justifiable. Winning is only part of the game. One should not concentrate on winning at any cost, regardless of how the game is played (by fair means or foul). As long as the game is played according to predetermined rules acceptable to all the participants, fair play should lead to the best outcome for all.

When you apply this overriding principle to decision-making situations, it is apparent that some well-considered decisions will not pan out as expected.

19. Why do we regret decisions that did not 'succeed'?

Look back and recall how the decision was made. If you did your 'homework' carefully, diligently and in good faith, and yet the decision ended up as a 'failure,' don't blame yourself. This happens. It is a game of probability. Many factors (attributable to chance) may have intervened to prevent the expected outcome. It is a good idea to find out what actually happened, why, and learn from that experience.

20. My heart says "Do," but my brain says "Don't." I am confused. What should I do?

This is common, when unresolved conflicts—hidden or apparent— loom in the background, nagging you. Your logical (thinking) brain may be warning you that the decision is not in your best interests. It pays to heed this 'yellow' warning signal and revisit the issue carefully. Also, your emotions (heart) and reason (brain) are not in sync when this happens—so be careful, exercise proper judgment before taking action. It is time to reflect and decide with a clear conscience, after having resolved the dilemma to your satisfaction.

21. What should I do when my spouse does not go along with my decision?

Marital harmony and mutual respect should inform family decisions. When this condition is absent, misunderstanding and discord will ensue. It is best to iron out the issues, negotiate, respect the other person's point of view, and come to a mutually agreeable solution, so that everyone involved can live with the proposed solution. If the issue at hand is especially important to one party, the other person may be willing to concede, provided he/she gets to do what 'they want' on another issue.

22. Are there 'shortcuts' to some decisions? Can the process be simplified?

Thankfully, yes. There are certain 'rules of thumb' that can be handy. These well-established dictums, discovered through personal or common human experience, can become useful in many situations. It is best to ask yourself whether they might be of help in your situation.

Here are some examples:

a. For those who seek safety and dislike taking risk: "A bird in the hand is worth two in the bush."

b. Saving for retirement: "Save at least 10% of your gross income: pay yourself first."

c. Forgiveness: "With malice toward none, and charity for all."

d. The principle of Occam's Razor: 'Practice simplicity.' "You don't need a shotgun to kill a mosquito."

e. Monthly mortgage payment should not exceed one-third of your income; total debt-service should be below 40%.

f. Heed these warnings; ignore them at your own peril:
"Investigate before you invest."
"If it is too good to be true, it probably is."
"A fool and his money are easily parted."

23. How can I align my habits with my decisions? They seem to be working at cross purposes.

This is a common problem. Habits, established over long periods of time, can stand in the way of implementing well-thought-out decisions. As a result, the decisions are aborted, ignored, or simply forgotten. The overriding force of habit can prevent 'good decisions' from being implemented. For example, New Year's resolutions such as:

I will start an exercise regimen or a new diet program to lose weight.

I will start saving for retirement starting next birthday.

I will drive carefully and avoid texting while doing so.

Good intentions are not enough to implement what you want to do. The force of 'bad habits' should not be underestimated; they can exercise their 'veto' power overriding your decisions. This is akin to working against 'gravity.' It is a battle which is worth fighting for and winning. Right now, they are exercising their relentless mastery over you and declaring victory! Your dogged determination, perseverance, and strong sense of purpose must be marshalled against these stubborn 'enemies,' if you want to win this battle. It is up to you to choose—win or lose!

24. What if I made a 'bad' decision, which I now regret? What should be done to repair the damage?

    i.   This is all too common. You had the good sense to admit your mistake. That is to be applauded.

    ii.   If the 'damage' can be repaired, please take remedial action as soon as possible.

    iii.   If you have unwittingly hurt someone, ask for their forgiveness and offer to compensate.

iv. This is a great opportunity for you to learn from your mistake; ask yourself: 'What lesson can I derive from this unfortunate episode?'

25. People say that I decide hastily and end up making poor decisions. What can I do to make better decisions? Is there a formula that can be applied? How can I educate myself on this subject?

You can take many steps to improve your performance.

A. Think clearly about the issue at hand.

B. Collect all relevant facts and make sure they are timely and reliable.

C. Have a good grip on your priorities and set an achievable goal.

D. Try to balance 'hasty, emotional, gut reactions' with logical analysis.

E. Look at all available options; study each one carefully.

F. Conduct a thorough cost-benefit analysis of the best available option.

G. Put sufficient resources—time, energy, money and skills—behind your preferred solution.

H. Implement the decision wholeheartedly; monitor it and wait for results.

I. Accept the consequences whatever they are; take responsibility for the outcome.

J. Learn from this experience, to help prepare for the next challenge.

Post-Mortem

Here is an exercise to review how satisfied/dissatisfied you were with a major decision you made during the past six months. Recall the circumstances surrounding the decision. When you made the decision, you were concerned with improving some aspect of your life. Now is an opportune time to look back and evaluate the 'quality' of that decision, based on all the criteria governing a well-thought-out decision (discussed in this book).

1. In what way was this decision significant?
2. How was it designed to improve your quality of life? Did you foresee how it might turn out?
3. Did you do a thorough CBA of all the options available to you?
4. Did you have enough time to think and plan what you wanted to do? Was the decision undertaken after conducting 'due diligence'?
5. Hypothetically, could a decision not to proceed with the chosen option reduce your overall wellbeing?
6. With the benefit of hindsight, would you make the same decision? If so, why? If not, why not? How would you modify it in any way?
7. Did you implement the decision wholeheartedly? Were there unanticipated difficulties/glitches in doing so?
8. Has the decision worked out to your satisfaction? How have you benefited from it? Have the results exceeded your expectations or fallen short? Explain clearly, and if possible, in quantitative terms.
9. Did the expected benefits justify the associated costs? Which of those benefits failed to materialize?

10. Faced with the same circumstances, how would you do things differently now (if at all)? What does this say about your pre-decision state of mind?

This type of 'post-mortem' analysis can help to understand why you did what you did—and more importantly, given the same pre-decision circumstances, how might you do anything differently now. If you face a similar situation in the future, can you make a 'better' decision? What useful lessons did you learn from your previous experience?

Ode to Decision Making

Carefully analyze and evaluate all relevant issues.
Ponder appropriate steps needed to solve the problem.
Take account of all potential costs and benefits.
Consider a long-term plan rather than just immediate prospects.
Be empathetic, humble and know your limitations.
Use your intuition to know what will work and what will not.
Use experience to throw light on the current situation.
Examine the issue from different perspectives and angles.
Have consideration for others and their points of view.
Respect how others react to your suggestions and opinions.
Seek advice and input from experts whenever necessary.
Don't pretend you know all the answers.
Control your emotions and do not be carried away by them.
Be able to evaluate what is relevant and what is not.
Learn to separate 'wheat from chaff.'
Cultivate judgment, perception and ability to separate fact from fiction.
Do not fall prey to temptation, false promises or bribery
Know your mind and have clarity of vision.
Adhere to the truth, have integrity, and keep your word.

Some Parting Words

I sincerely hope that readers will benefit from the wealth of ideas, examples, anecdotes and case studies presented here. Their sole purpose is to instruct, inform, educate and entertain. Depending on one's needs and inclinations, you may (or may not) find them appropriate and suitable in your decision-making. As explained earlier, there is no guarantee that any single decision strategy will result in producing the expected outcomes. Remember: Both choice and chance play their respective roles in the game of life.

The author welcomes your comments and suggestions.

Please write to:

patha1934@gmail.com or

doraig@wpunj.edu

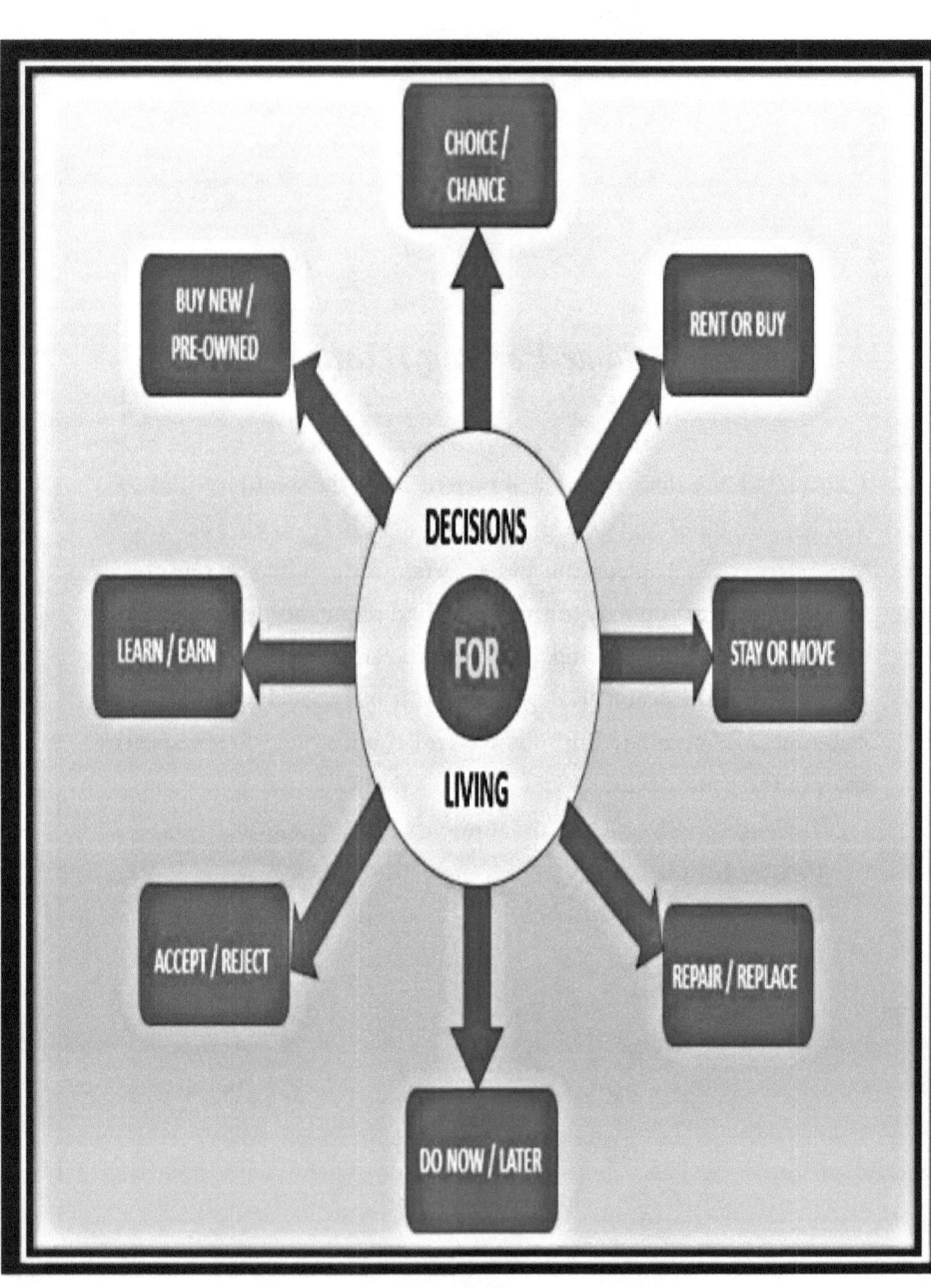

Index